"The development in thinking and practice of neuroscience is exciting for a number of reasons, not the least because of its impact on the arts therapies. This book contains a treasure trove of writing, encompassing the work of a variety of creative arts practitioners, and is inspiring and uplifting. Music, art, movement and drama are combined in this unique text which contains a veritable treasure trove of writing exploring the benefits of creative therapeutic work for a wide range of clients. The book also provides an opportunity to hear different voices from the global practices of these creative therapists, adding much to the discourse and practice development for colleagues in a variety of fields as well as students and those with lived-experience of the life-issues presented here."

– **Dr Elizabeth Coombes,** *FHEA FAMI. Therapydd Cerdd/Music Therapist, Uwch Ddarlithydd/Senior Lecturer, Arweinydd Rhaglen MA mewn Therapi Cerdd/Programme Leader MA Music Therapy, Rhoelwr Academaidd/Academic Manager, Prifysgol De Cymru/University of South Wales*

"The arts therapies are uniquely positioned to contribute significantly to the practical and experiential applications of recent developments in neuroscience to mental health. Arts therapists have long practiced with a deep understanding of the connection between mind and body. This volume is an eloquent contribution to this field and ensures that the experience and understanding of the arts therapists is heard and included. It is especially exciting to hear the stories and experiences of arts therapists who bring their experience from beyond the global North."

– **Paula Kingwill,** *Dramatherapist, HPCSA reg. South Africa*

"An extraordinary culmination of innovative and captivating practice and insights from a diverse cross-section of international arts therapies practitioners and contexts. Each chapter sensitively considers the complexities of neuroscience, how emerging research is stimulating engagement with the arts and creativity across the lifespan, and how these implications are impacting informed practice. Those receiving arts therapies services remain the focal point and it is their engagement with the creative processes that breathe life into the discourse. Caroline Miller has again contributed a critical and sophisticated text that interweaves theory, research, and neuroscience that is sure to ignite your imagination and progress the arts therapies in important ways."

– **Ronald P.M.H. Lay,** *MA, AThR, ATR-BC, registered and credentialed art therapist, consultant, supervisor and program leader of the Masters in Art Therapy Program at LASALLE College of the Arts, Singapore*

"This very readable, enriching and enlightening book contains chapters from Arts Therapists who practice in a range of continents, with a wide variety of clients. Each writer provides an engaging case study to illustrate how a synthesis of theories from the arts, science and psychotherapy combined with humanity informs their approaches to therapy."

– **Madeline Andersen-Warren,** *author, researcher and recently retired dramatherapist, UK*

"Many people imagine that the arts have a profound effect on the body, mind and psyche. The authors in this book argue that these benefits can be explained through better understanding of neuroscience. From drama to dance and music, through arts and the imagination, multiple stories unfold here to pique the reader's curiosity and help them envisage the relationship between the arts and neurological change."

– **Prof Katrina Skewes McFerran,** *The University of Melbourne, Australia*

Arts Therapies in International Practice

Arts Therapies in International Practice: Informed by Neuroscience and Research brings together practice and research in the arts therapies and in neuroscience. The authors are all arts therapists who have reviewed their practice through the lens of modern neuroscience. Neuroscience confirms the importance of embodiment, choice, and creativity in therapy with a range of clients. Arts therapies directly provide these.

The authors demonstrate how the arts therapies can be adapted creatively to work in different social and ethnic communities, with different ages and with different states of health or ill health. Although there is diversity in their practice and country of practice, they reaffirm key concepts of the arts therapies, such as the importance of the therapeutic relationship, and the key role played by the arts modality with its effects on the brain and nervous system.

This book will appeal to a wide readership, including arts therapists, expressive arts therapists, a range of other psychotherapists and counsellors, students and their teachers, and those interested in the neuroscience of human development.

Caroline Miller, (NZ) MA Clinical Psychology, PGDip Clinical Psychology, BA English/Psychology, BPhil, PG Dip. Dramatherapy, graduated as a dramatherapist in 1991 and has worked as a dramatherapist and clinical psychologist in government services, non-government services, schools, mental health settings, and private practice. Her work has included school counselling, managing and setting up a district health board mental health service for children adolescents and their families, managing a programme for conduct disordered youth, working in schools for children (ages 5–21) with special needs, working with young sex offenders, and working in private practice with adults and young people with sexual abuse trauma, depression, anxiety, and other diagnosed mental health disorders. She has had an extensive supervision practice. She has supported many therapists to develop their writing for publication. Caroline was the inaugural co-director of the MA in arts therapy, a combined arts therapies programme at Whitecliffe College of Arts and Design in Auckland New Zealand. She continued in the position of co-director teaching and supervising master's-level dissertations. This was followed by guest lecturing and workshop invitations. She has presented at several conferences in Australasia and the United Kingdom. Caroline has published several articles and is the editor of two books *Assessment and Outcomes in the Arts Therapies: A Person-Centred Approach* (London, UK: Jessica Kingsley Publishers, 2014), and *Arts Therapists in Multidisciplinary Settings: Working Together for Better Outcomes* (London, UK: Jessica Kingsley Publishers, 2016).

Mariana Torkington, (NZ) MA Arts Therapy (Clinical), AThR, ANZACATA, MNZAC, ACC Provider, is a registered arts therapist working and lecturing in Auckland and a published author in the arts therapies field. Mariana has worked as an arts therapist for government and non-government agencies and in private practice. She has specialised in working with children, adolescents and families in trauma and abuse recovery. Her special areas of interest include family work, learning disabilities, anxiety, and depression. Mariana is currently lecturing in the newly established Child and Adolescent Psychotherapy Programme at Auckland University of Technology. Mariana spent her childhood and young adulthood living in Argentina and Brazil and speaks Spanish, Portuguese, and English.

Arts Therapies in International Practice

Informed by Neuroscience and Research

Edited by Caroline Miller and Mariana Torkington

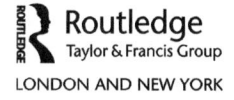

LONDON AND NEW YORK

First published 2022
by Routledge
2 Park Square, Milton Park, Abingdon, Oxon OX14 4RN

and by Routledge
605 Third Avenue, New York, NY 10158

Routledge is an imprint of the Taylor & Francis Group, an informa business

British Library Cataloguing-in-Publication Data
A catalogue record for this book is available from the British Library

Library of Congress Cataloging-in-Publication Data
Names: Miller, Caroline (Clinical psychologist), editor. | Torkington, Mariana, editor.
Title: Arts therapies in international practice: informed by neuroscience and research / edited by Caroline Miller and Mariana Torkington.
Description: Milton Park, Abingdon, Oxon ; New York, NY: Routledge, 2022. | Includes bibliographical references and index. |
Identifiers: LCCN 2021037469 | ISBN 9780367536862 (hardback) | ISBN 9780367536886 (paperback) | ISBN 9781003082897 (ebook)
Subjects: LCSH: Art therapy.
Classification: LCC RC489.A7 A774 2022 | DDC 616.89/1656—dc23
LC record available at https://lccn.loc.gov/2021037469

ISBN: 978-0-367-53686-2 (hbk)
ISBN: 978-0-367-53688-6 (pbk)
ISBN: 978-1-003-08289-7 (ebk)

DOI: 10.4324/9781003082897

Typeset in Bembo
by Apex CoVantage, LLC

Contents

Figures

Chapter 3

Chapter 5

Chapter 6

Chapter 7

Chapter 8

Chapter 10

Contributors' bios

Vanitha Chandrasegaram, (Malaysia), MA Dramatherapy, UK; MSc Psychology, USA; Member of NADTA, USA, is a pioneer dramatherapist in Malaysia. She has 14 years of experience practising dramatherapy in settings such as psychiatric hospitals and wards, non-government organisations, and universities. She has conducted dramatherapy skills training sessions in Australia, Lebanon, India, and Malaysia. Her experience includes working with individuals and groups who have experience of abuse, learning disabilities, mental health problems, emotional difficulties, relationship challenges, and other life challenges. She has worked with individuals and groups with ages ranging from 3 to 90 years old. She has headed a home for more than 70 underprivileged children from ages 4 to 16. Vanitha has presented at conferences and facilitated workshops/training in the United Kingdom, the United States, India, Lebanon, Australia, and Iceland. Her work has been published in professional journals in the United Kingdom. She has also lectured at colleges and universities and taught theatre for seniors for the U3A (University of the Third Age). Her interests include dancing, acting, and playing the flute. She is a certified yoga instructor.

Verity Danbold (Dance Therapy Association of Australasia [DTAA], ADM-PUK, MNCP, Accred.) (Australia), is a dance movement therapist (DMT) specialising in trauma. As both a dance movement therapist (DMT certification, Kolkata Sanved/TISS Mumbai) and a community theatre dance/social circus specialist (MA Theatre and Development, University of East Anglia), she has extensive experience working globally with refugees and survivors of sex trafficking, child marriage, and torture. She was a Hanny Exiner Memorial Fellow for the DTAA. She currently works with young survivors of sexual abuse in the United Kingdom.

DMT uses movement as a diagnostic and healing tool, seeing in the body what Ruth St Denis described as "too fine, too deep" for words. She draws from the Sampoornata method, a human-rights based methodology, and campaigns for client rights outside of sessions, while holding a creative, nurturing space for clients to grow as their own advocate. She guides her practice as one of "working through the body what is done to the body".

Working in the global South for over a decade, she celebrates the capacity for movement to transcend cultural and language barriers and to connect with non/pre-verbal clients. She integrates practices such as circus, yoga, and crafts to celebrate the creative, reflective, and moving self. In working through the body and movement, she nurtures a practice of body-embedded self-care, encouraging people to reflect on themselves as a tool for healing, strength, and growth.

Agnès Desombiaux-Sigley (New Zealand) was educated in France in French and European philosophical and analytical traditions. This forms the background to her approach to psychodynamic art psychotherapy. She offers her clients a wide range of art materials in each session. Through her training in sand play therapy, symbol work, and multimodal arts therapy, she provides opportunities for her clients to work more clearly with projection and with externalisation of situations. From further training and experience of somatic therapy with trauma, she has developed a greater awareness of the physical sensations experienced by her clients as they work through trauma experiences and the consequences of these. More recently, she has been developing awareness of the physical sensations she experiences while working with clients. She reflects on these as mirrors to the clients' psychic and somatic experiences in the present. Agnès is an arts therapist, AThR, and a psychotherapist. She has a PG Diploma in Health Science (expressive therapies), PG Certif. Psychosomatic Integration Treatment (PSI Institute), PG Cert. Family Therapy (NZAFT), PG Cert. Sand Play Therapy and Symbol Work and Proficiency in the Treaty of Waitangi, BA Communication. She holds professional registration with the Australia, New Zealand, and Asian Creative Arts Therapies Association; New Zealand Association of Psychotherapists (provisional); New Zealand Association of Family Therapy (clinical member); and Waka Oranga (National Collective of Maori Psychotherapy Practitioners, associate member). She works with children, youth, and adults in private practice (in English and French) in central Auckland. She is contracted by Accident Compensation Corporation (ACC), a government agency which funds counselling services for survivors of sexual abuse. Agnès is a published author and has presented at international conferences.

Renda Dionne Madrigal, PhD (USA, Turtle Mountain Chippewa) is a licensed clinical psychologist, UCLA Certified Mindfulness Facilitator, registered dramatherapist, Narradrama facilitator, somatic experiencing practitioner, and member of the Turtle Mountain Band of Chippewa Indians. She is the author of *The Mindful Family Guidebook* (PenguinRandomHouse.com, 2021). She was featured on the cover of the February 2018 edition of *Mindful Magazine*. She has been a licensed clinical psychologist for more than 25 years. She is also a teaching assistant/advisor for the UCLA Mindfulness Awareness Research Center, partner of the Cousins Center for Psychoneuroimmunology within the Semel Institute for Neuroscience and Human Behavior, Teacher Training Program. She has served as co-investigator on three National Institute of Drug Abuse-funded prevention projects within the Native American community, as a consultant for the University of California Davis Resource Center for Family Focused Practice, and for Riverside Department of Public Social Services and Riverside University Health Systems on engaging tribes in wellness. She was one of the steering team members for a project funded by the Children's Bureau for Bringing and Building Evidence in the Child Welfare System. She has also served as an associate research scientist with the Oregon Research Institute. She has presented at numerous conferences and trainings at the tribal, county, state, and federal levels. She has been involved in a Therapeutic Theatre Project, *Menil and Her Heart and Wildflower Indigenous Spirit*. In her clinical practice, she utilizes mindfulness, somatic experiencing (body-based), and creative arts (Narradrama, dramatherapy, and storytelling) as healing modalities. She is the president of Mindful Practice Inc. and faculty at the Drama Therapy Institute of Los Angeles and at California Indian Nations College.

Pamela Dunne, PhD, RDT/BCT (USA), is a registered dramatherapist, board-certified trainer, psychologist, and professor emerita at California State University Los Angeles and Executive Director of the Drama Therapy Institute of Los Angeles (DTILA). The Institute was established in 1990 as an approved alternative training program by the North American Drama Therapy Association (NADTA). Dr Dunne also directs the Creative Therapy Center, which offers psychotherapy services and support groups for Southern California. Dr Dunne is the author of well over a dozen books, films, articles, and book chapters. She has offered training worldwide. For over 14 years, under her leadership the DTILA has offered an annual summer abroad program, conducting drama therapy training and workshops in Europe and Great Britain from Greece to Stockholm to Ireland, with a programme centred on Narradrama and creative arts. Dr Dunne has pioneered dramatherapy and Narradrama training in China and Russia. She is past president of the NADTA and past founding board member of the Drama Therapy Fund. In 2014, she was honoured to receive the Teaching Excellence Award in recognition of her outstanding dedication to education in the field of drama therapy through teaching and mentorship given by the NADTA. In 2016, the NADTA presented her with the Gertrud Schattner Award for outstanding achievement in Drama Therapy. In 2018 she was one of the keynote speakers and workshop leaders for the first International Drama Therapy Conference in China in Beijing.

Kim Hau Pang, MA, AThR (Singapore), holds a Master of Arts Art Therapy from LASALLE College of the Arts Singapore after graduating with a BA (Hons) Fine Art from Loughborough University, United Kingdom. He is credentialed through the Australian, New Zealand and Asian Creative Arts Therapies Association and is a professional member with the Art Therapists' Association Singapore. Pang has presented his work at international art therapy conferences in Australia and the United Kingdom; and is a contributing author for *Found Objects in Art Therapy: Materials and Process* (Jessica Kings-ley, 2021). His art practice had led to his solo exhibition *Unplanned End-ings* (2019) at Intersections Art Gallery in Singapore, with the support from National Arts Council (Singapore). Pang's art installations have also been presented in arts and cultural institutions such as the *Singapore Art Museum* (2017), *Owl Spot Theatre* in Tokyo, Japan (2016 and 2017), and, most recently, *The Herbert Art Gallery & Museum* in Coventry, United King-dom (2021). He is currently practising as an art therapist at Assisi Hospice, Singapore.

Sarah Mann Shaw (UK) is a dramatherapist and psychotherapist in private practice. She has a PG. Dipl. in Dramatherapy from Hertfordshire Col-lege of Art and Design, MA in Integrative Psychotherapy, Diploma in Life Coaching, and Diploma in Psychotherapy with Children and Young Peo-ple. She has extensive experience working with children and adolescents alongside statutory and private agencies. She works with the impact of dis-rupted attachments and trauma using dramatherapy. Sarah has been inte-grating theories of neuroscience into her work for many years and finds it a particularly helpful addition to her work. Sarah has contributed to *Drama as Therapy, Theory, Practice, Research*, vol. 2 (Routledge, 2007), written a chap-ter for *Routledge International Handbook of Dramatherapy* (2016) and has two articles published in the *Dramatherapy Journal*, 'Metaphor, symbol and the healing process in Dramatherapy' (1996, vol. 18, no 2, pp. 2–5), and 'The drama of shame', co-written with Di Gammage (November 2011, vol. 33, pp. 131–143).

Caroline Miller, (NZ) MA Clinical Psychology, PGDip Clinical Psychol-ogy, BA English/Psychology, BPhil, PG Dip. Dramatherapy, graduated as a dramatherapist in 1991 and has worked as a dramatherapist and clinical psy-chologist in government services, non-government services, schools, mental health settings, and in private practice. Her work has included school coun-selling, managing and setting up a District Health Board mental health ser-vice for children adolescents and their families, managing a programme for conduct-disordered youth, working in schools for children (ages 5–21) with special needs, working with young sex offenders, and working in private practice with adults and young people with sexual abuse trauma, depression, anxiety, and other diagnosed mental health disorders. She has had exten-sive supervision practice. She has supported many therapists to develop their writing for publication. Caroline was the inaugural co-director of the MA in Arts Therapy, a combined arts therapies programme at Whitecliffe College of Arts and Design in Auckland, New Zealand. She continued in the position of co-director teaching and supervising master's-level disserta-tions. This was followed by guest lecturer and workshop invitations. She has presented at several conferences in Australasia and the United Kingdom. Caroline has published several articles and is the editor of two books, *Assess-ment and Outcomes in the Arts Therapies: A Person-Centred Approach* (London,

UK: Jessica Kingsley Publishers, 2014) and *Arts Therapists in Multidisciplinary Settings: Working Together for Better Outcomes* (London, UK: Jessica Kingsley Publishers, 2016).

Sian Palmer (South Africa) graduated in Drama and Movement Therapy (MA) with Distinction from the Royal Central School of Speech Drama, University of London, in 2009. On completing her studies, Sian returned to Johannesburg, South Africa, where she started Expressive Movement open classes and opened her private practice as a drama therapist. The development of the Expressive Movement form was informed by the Laban and Movement with Touch strands of the Sesame approach to drama and movement therapy, Jungian theory, and Sian's years of experience in contemporary and conscious dance. Since 2015, Sian has trained 34 facilitators of Expressive Movement across South Africa. Sian spent seven years as lead Trainer of the Firemaker Project with the Zakheni Arts Therapy Foundation, training social workers and care workers in building resilience through integrating the creative arts into their psychosocial support groups with children and young people. Pioneering the field of dramatherapy in South Africa, Sian was head lecturer on the first dramatherapy training in Africa at Wits University, leading the Introduction to Drama Therapy Course and Honours Drama Therapy Programme from 2014 to 2016. Following training in Family Constellations in 2015, she co-founded a systemic approach, Ancestral Connections, with clinical psychologist and Family Constellations Trainer, Tanja Meyburgh. Ancestral Connections integrates Expressive Movement and constellations practice. Since 2009, Sian's clinical practice in dramatherapy has included working in schools and privately with children with special needs, young people with emotional and behavioural difficulties, and adults living with mental health issues including bipolar disorder, depression, and anxiety. With her area of expertise firmly established in embodied practice, Sian is passionate about a holistic approach to healing and growth, recognising the importance of connecting with our roots and ancestral lineages, being in community, connecting with nature as a resource, and tapping into our innate creativity.

Daphne Rickson is an adjunct professor at the New Zealand School of Music – Te Kōkī, Victoria University of Wellington, New Zealand. She has extensive experience as a music therapy practitioner, teacher, and researcher and is particularly renowned for her work with children and adolescents who have learning support needs. During her 17-year teaching career Daphne has taught and examined more than 100 postgraduate students and has given many international lectures. She maintains a sustained platform of internationally recognised research which focuses on music therapy to maximise the participation, inclusion, and wellbeing of diverse learners in schools and tertiary institutions, and the well-being of school communities generally. Her research has attracted significant external grants, led to invitations to speak at international conferences and to serve on scientific committees, and resulted in an extensive publication record, including 35 journal articles. She is also the co-author, with Katrina Skews McFerran, of the text *Creating Music Cultures in the Schools: A Perspective From Community Music Therapy* (Barcelona Publishers, 2014). Daphne is the current Australasian Regional Liaison on the World Federation of Music Therapy Council, and President Emeritus, and a Life Member, of Music Therapy New Zealand.

Alison Talmage, MEd, MMusTher, PhD candidate (New Zealand), completed her music therapy training at the New Zealand School of Music, Wellington, studying with Robert Krout, Daphne Rickson, and Sarah Hoskyns. She is currently a doctoral student at the University of Auckland, supervised by Dr Te Oti Rakena, Professor Suzanne Purdy, and Adjunct Professor Daphne Rickson. Alison's eclectic music therapy practice draws on clinical, community, and interdisciplinary frameworks; neuroscience and speech science research; and the holistic biopsychosocial-spiritual approach. Her current practice and research focus on the CeleBRation Choir at the University of Auckland's Centre for Brain Research (CBR) and Sing Up Rodney, a community music therapy group administered by the Kahikatea Music Therapy and Community Arts Trust. Both groups offer therapeutic community singing for adults who have neurogenic communication difficulties resulting from an acquired neurological condition, such as stroke, aphasia, Parkinson's disease, dementia, or traumatic brain injury. Alison's doctoral action research study focuses on the improvement of practice, the relationship between research and professional practice, and professional and stakeholder perspectives. Alison is the editor of the *New Zealand Journal of Music Therapy*; the coordinator of the CBR Neurological Singing, Choir and Voice Network; and the coordinator of the Music Therapy New Zealand Research Special Interest Group.

Mariana Torkington, MA Arts Therapy (Clinical), AThR, ANZACATA, MNZAC, ACC Provider (New Zealand), is a registered arts therapist working and lecturing in Auckland, and a published author in the arts therapies field. Her publications include chapters in arts therapies books, articles, and images in journals and edited books. Mariana has worked as an arts therapist for government and non-government agencies and in private practice. She has specialised in working with children, adolescents and families in trauma and abuse recovery. Her special areas of interest include family work, learning disabilities, anxiety, and depression. Mariana is currently lecturing in the newly established Child and Adolescent Psychotherapy Programme at Auckland University of Technology and running a small private practice. Mariana and Bruce Torkington are responsible for all the images and other graphics in this book. Mariana spent her childhood and young adulthood living in Argentina and Brazil and speaks Spanish, Portuguese, and English.

Foreword: a treatise for change

Noah Hass-Cohen

The broad range of expressive arts approaches described in this publication are compelling examples of how international expressive arts therapists have taken innovative steps to take advantage of the abundance of information from clinical neuroscience research (Hass-Cohen, 2008). Findings from neuroscience have suggested that the arts in psychotherapy provide unique advantages for recovery and resiliency (Hass-Cohen, 2016). Co-editor Caroline Miller has persuasively compiled, in the first chapter, a contemporary selection and description of such advances. Indeed, in this internationally focused publication, authors have exquisitely described how they have utilised and integrated the unique neuroscience-based aspects of the arts in psychotherapy to further our field. They are to be applauded for their theoretical and pragmatic contributions. Given my background, I am particularly honoured to join this international group of neuroscience-committed art therapists. Originally from Israel, I have lived in Los Angeles for a little over three decades. Like many of the authors, I had to proactively seek out training and learning about these neuroscientific endeavours. One of my endeavours has been to provide a theoretical frame for an Art Therapy Relational Neuroscience (ATR-N) approach (Hass-Cohen & Clyde Findlay, 2015). From a neuropsychological perspective, memory recall and reconsolidation are unifying psychotherapy agents of change. The therapeutic utilisation of ATR-N principles has a key role in positively scaffolding and sequencing memory reconsolidation (MR) processes (Hass-Cohen et al., 2014, 2018; Hass-Cohen & Clyde Findlay, 2019).

The ATR-N principles are represented by the acronym CREATE: (a) Creative Embodiment, specifically creativity, pleasure imagination, and movement; (b) Relational Resonating, specifically the therapeutic relationship; (c) Expressive Communicating, specifically utilising diverse arts psychotherapies modalities; (d) Adaptive Responding, specifically perceived safeness, comfort, and internal and external locus of executive control; and (e) Empathising and Compassion, specifically enhanced by the functions of mirror neurons systems, positive emotions, gratitude, and kindness (Hass-Cohen & Clyde Findlay, 2015).

MR and the expressive arts in psychotherapy

As distressing and arousing memories arise and are recalled and processed, they ideally fade or integrate into autobiographical and semantic memory. Memories guide the interpersonal sense of self, actions, and plans; we like to think that they are lasting and stable. In fact, memories are not "forever". Neuroscientific evidence suggests that memories become fluid during remembrance and vulnerable to either reinforcement or to reconsolidation and change (Schwabe et al., 2014). Reinforcement runs the risk of retraumatisation. For about four to six hours after the recollection, proteins in the fear and memory centres of the brain (the lateral amygdala and the hippocampus) break down until they resynthesise in the hippocampus (Nader et al., 2000; LeDoux, 2000). Thus, it is possible to modify autobiographical memories by positive responses during this window of opportunity. This process reoccurs with any memory recall (Nader et al., 2000; Tronson & Taylor, 2007) and most likely in every psychotherapy session.

MR requires the sequencing of strategic conditions (Hass-Cohen, 2018; Hass-Cohen & Clyde-Findlay, 2019; Simon et al., 2020). The recall of the trauma memory, the reminder, must be short and followed by new knowledge (Lane et al., 2015). This situation happens easily in the arts psychotherapy as immediately after the client shares the problem memory, we shift into engagement with new experiences of the arts activities. Conversely, while engaging in the expressive arts-making may inadvertently briefly trigger a reminder of the trauma, artmaking simultaneously securely anchors the distress in a creative container.

After the reminder (or concurrently), the memory must be disturbed by a prediction error; otherwise, the original memory is reinforced (Lane et al., 2015), posing a risk for retraumatisation. When there is a mismatch between what is expected and what happens a prediction error happens, this pairing between old memories and new events continues to destabilise the memory (Lee et al., 2017). In psychotherapy, negatively loaded memories would ideally be matched with unexpected positive or disconfirming loaded experiences (Ecker et al., 2015; Schiller, 2010). Therapeutic strategies such as contextual processing (Brewin, 2018; Hupbach et al., 2008) decrease the re-experiencing of perceived inescapable flashbacks and trauma (Hartley et al., 2014). The aims are to successfully dislodge the impact of negative self-beliefs, -biases, and -appraisals (Agren, 2014; Brewin, 2018). Acknowledging here and now safety destabilises the hold of a threatening memory while focusing on creating a contingent, coherent, and organised recall further contextualizes autobiographical memories. Examples include the therapist's validating responses, examination of the validity of negative self-bias or the necessity of problem maintenance. Accessing related positive explicit memories is critical to supportive MR as otherwise fear-based memories are unfortunately strengthened (Barreiro et al., 2013).

Both implicit and explicit expressive arts practices innately provide this mismatch. Revisiting fear-based memories with optimism and hope-based creative learning are some of the strategies that arts-based therapies use to place fear in the past. To do so, interventions must trigger cognitive surprise, curiosity, and attention (Wichert et al., 2013) and support meaning-making (Hupbach, 2011). The ability to generate vivid mental imagery positive future events may provide is an MR factor. For example, the vividness of positive future imagery was significantly associated with optimism (Murphy et al., 2015). Other examples include the juxtaposition of the joy of creation, or neutral procedural art-based skills with an avoidant reaction. Fortuitously, arts-based sensory cues, that is visual, iconic, auditory, olfactory, and spatial experiences seem to effectively assist in the updating of existing memories. However, habitual negative reactions may interfere with successful memory modulation. This retroactive interference is less likely to occur when MR processes are prompted by non-verbal arts modalities, namely sensory, visual, and spatial interventions (Fougnie & Marois, 2011). Likely due to the hippocampal memory centre's vulnerability to such clues and additional storage capacity for sensory information (Luck & Vogel, 2013), the phenomenon speaks to the advantages of the arts-based psychotherapies. These MR strategies lead to lasting resiliency and recovery (De Gauna et al., 2015).

CREATE memory reconsolidation strategies

Creative Embodiment is at the core of expressive drama and dance therapies. Kinaesthetic movement functions in the processing of insecure memory and likely MR (Silva & Soares, 2018). In her chapter, Sian Palmer describes how community dancing at a women's conference in Johannesburg, South Africa, instilled a secure base of support. Citing interpersonal neurobiology literature, she describes how rhythmic dancing in a circle created opportunities to repair feelings of insecurity by mismatching traumatic memories with being seen and accepted by others. Verity Danbold further extrapolates on the universal and culturally shared advantages of dance therapy. She helps us understand that dancing should not be interpreted formally, but rather, it should be globally conceptualised as creative movement that embodies empathic social interactions. Verity Danbold also reminds us that motor activity has the potential to access trauma that is stored in the body while at the same time providing an opportunity to turn to others and befriend rather than fight, hide, or freeze (Taylor, 2006). The dance therapy advantages that the authors discuss are scaffolded by relational resonating and adaptive responding treatment principles.

Relational Resonance ATR-N strategies are critical mediators of memory recall and reconsolidation. From infancy throughout the life span, the social brain uniquely engages people in continuous efforts to express and dampen, that is self-regulate, emotional experiences. Multiple neural subcortical, limbic, and cortical pathways are involved (Hass-Cohen & Carr, 2008). These integrative nervous system functions transform sensory and emotive bottom-up expression and cortical top-down regulation of affect (Baumeister & Vohs, 2004). Important in these efforts is the activation of the ventral arm of the polyvagal system which is initiated during soft, warm, and tender relationships (Porges, 2001). Sarah Mann Shaw's chapter on attachment and dramatherapy provides a compelling example of how the arts may stimulate such vagal relational resonance. Embodied dramatised play (Jennings, 2011) is a way to access shared implicit metaphors to fully engage the mother and child in a reparative bond.

Music therapy provides a unique verbal and non-verbal approach to polyvagal activation (Porges et al., 2014). It is in this vein that Daphne Rickson describes the interpersonal neuroscience research related to her work with children with autism. Specific gains include emotional regulation, intrapersonal and interpersonal regulation, and an increased ability to engage socially and share with others. Daphne Rickson illustrates her approach with a case study while continuing to advocate for additional research. It is likely that in the presence of an affectionate therapeutic relationship, texture, touch, and movement of the ventral polyvagal support feelings of familiarity, bonding, and hopefulness (Porges, 2001).

Empathy and compassion are learned through the imitation and observation of another's actions, and importantly recognising that someone else's action is something that we can also do (Hass-Cohen, 2007; Gallese, 2003). In her chapter on dramatherapy with adolescents in Malaysia, Vanitha Chandrasegaram clearly delineates how dramatherapy techniques activate mirroring systems in the nervous system and illuminates the connection between the arousal of social connectivity and the bonding neurochemical oxytocin. It is likely that in anticipation of the therapist's hands purposefully offering materials, demonstrating a movement, or encouraging playing, our clients' motor mirror neurons respond in kind, thereby creating deep engagements: "I can do what you do, and feel what you feel" (Hass-Cohen & Clyde Findlay, 2015).

Expressive communication provides a unique opportunity for taming traumatic aroused reactions. While colours, shapes, and symbols trigger emotionally rich limbic and poignant right hemispheric memories, the left hemisphere and higher prefrontal cortex areas plot to execute purposeful and tangible creations that calm the mind. Creativity, imagination, and the pleasure derived from arts-based sensory and mobile experiences contribute to the catecholamine-induced rewards and reduction of distress-based responses. In her chapter, Vanitha Chandrasegaram provides insights as to how mindful drama therapy techniques may further a sense of spatial control and have the potential to regulate stress-induced cortisol loops that have gone awry. When engaging in the arts, it is possible to address painful memories while experiencing internal and external loci of mastery and control (Hass-Cohen et al., 2020). Sensory experiences include touch, movement, visuals, and sound. Junctures where different areas in the brain meet, such as the sensory motor strip and the superior temporal gyrus, are areas of polymodal integration, suggesting that our brain has developed to effectively delight and make good use of sensory integration activities and kinaesthetic movement associated with expressive arts therapy activities. It is also critical to explicate that these efforts are scaffolded by the therapeutic alliance, again engaging the social engagement polyvagal ventral pathway (Hass-Cohen, 2016). This contrasts with verbally constrained therapy interventions that may not provide an escape hatch provided by involvement with arts (Kravits, 2008).

Expressive Communicating relates to stimulating emotional engagement within the art therapy environment. This emotional engagement is necessary for triggering meaningful MR reminders and potent prediction errors and likely charges the neurological reward circuitry while helping maintain a dynamic balance between excitation, pleasure, and tranquillity. Mariana Torkington (co-editor) discusses the role of imagination for trauma-informed arts psychotherapy. Beyond creativity, imagination is indeed a critical MR-related ingredient for two reasons. The first and foremost is for people to be able to imagine themselves speaking out without being retraumatised and experiencing further hurt. The second is for people to be able to visualise a different autobiographical memory ending that is devoid of ruptures and pain. In a similar vein, associating positive emotions expands people's horizons to access reliable reactions to problems (Fredrickson, 2013). In their research-based chapter, Pamela Dunne and Renda Dionne Madrigal demonstrate how their unique group-based Narradrama approach seeds, expands, and germinates new positive perspectives on distressing familiar narratives.

Alison Talmage describes how expressive communication, facilitated by singing in neurological choirs, can circumvent neurogenic communication challenges. She postulates that community singing in the CeleBRation Choir supports an updated autobiographical narrative by recruiting broad brain-based intrapersonal and interpersonal neuropathways that successfully compete for the same pathways that maintain the distressing memory. She explores how body language, facial expressions, and interpersonal space contribute to clinically observed positive effects and ends with a call for additional empirical studies.

Adaptive responding relies on the art therapist's capacity to provide an environment in which the client feels a degree of personal control, acceptance, resiliency, and safety. This is particularly helpful for trauma clients, as artmaking in this context can support the reframing of traumatic experiences and generates solutions. In her chapter, Agnès Desombiaux-Sigley adds to this clinical knowledge by providing an in-depth multimodal case study. She explains how the effects of generational grief and complex trauma are modulated and shaped into a recovered and coherent autobiographical sense of self. Therapeutically, a familiar therapeutic spatial location, such as the therapy space, may also support positive MR (Hupbach et al., 2008).

Kim Hau Pang writes about the Always Remembering Them program in a hospice setting in Singapore. He reminds us that across cultures it is incumbent on expressive arts therapists to engage in self-care as mirroring systems may contribute to therapist burnout and vicarious trauma associated with prolonged and uncontrolled stress responses. Undergoing stress, especially severe distress, places a persons' higher cognitive functions at risk, frequently leaving them without words to communicate and ask for support (Hull, 2002). Hence, it is essential for therapists to interact with non-verbal, emotion-based subcortical pathways (Schore, 2007) that frequently present as implicit imagery. This appreciation of the social and emotional role of the subcortical nervous system highlights the opportunities to receive therapeutic aid from the arts in psychotherapy whether in an individual or group format (Collie et al., 2006). Adaptive responses are contingent on one's actual and perceived sense of safety and are the most important change factors in psychotherapy (Hass-Cohen & Clyde Findlay, 2015).

Art psychotherapy provides people with enriching novel experiences which likely support brain plasticity. Under the right transformative and integrative conditions, neurons can regenerate in the memory centre of the brain (Eriksson et al., 1998; McEwen & Lasley, 2002) and perhaps even grow, leading to an increased capacity for autobiographical coherence. Accessing these implicit memory storages is easily facilitated by the arts psychotherapy as the memory centre of the brain is receptive to spatial cues and work. For example, hippocampal neurogenesis was noted during physical exercise in an enriched environment while learning new memory-based tasks (Colcombe et al., 2003; Elder et al., 2006). Hippocampal neurons tend to downregulate in reaction to chronic stressors such as grief (Bremner, 2006). The prefrontal lobes govern executive functions and an increased sense of internal and external locus of control. Moreover, achieving durable mental states entails integrating the left and right hemisphere functions (Schore, 2007; McNamee, 2003). Making art likely involves cognitive behavioral strategies that have been shown to change neural circuitry function (Lazar et al., 2005; Prasko et al., 2004; Straube et al., 2006), suggesting that artmaking, and subsequent meaning-making stimulate neurobiological changes (Hass-Cohen, 2016).

In summary, this treatise has argued that the CREATE ATR-principles support MR. This argument has the potential to organize a diverse body of art therapy approaches in a non-polemic way. From a neurobiological perspective, art-based sensory, perceptual, emotional, and cognitive processing mediate memory recall and reconsolidation and subsequent change. Thus, neuroscientific data provide us with a core foundation from which art therapists of any theoretical orientation can approach the interpersonal/felt aspects of art therapy. I would like to end by saluting and expressing my gratitude and appreciation for the expressive arts and neuroscientific contributions of the internal authors of this publication.

Biography

Dr. Noah Hass-Cohen is faculty at the Couple and Family Therapy program at Alliant International University in Los Angeles, California. She is an internationally recognised expert on relational art therapy neuroscience approaches. Noah is the author of two books, *Art Therapy & Clinical Neuroscience* and *Art Therapy & the Neuroscience of Relationships, Creativity & Resiliency*, which was published in Norton's Interpersonal Neuroscience series. She and a team of colleagues have received the prestigious *Journal of the American Art Therapy Association* article of the year research award for their trauma treatment case study in 2014. In 2019, she also received the prestigious Silver Rawley Research Grant from the American Art Therapy Association for her ongoing pain research. All her recent studies have focused on the application of her empirically supported four drawing protocol. Trained and certified in several mindfulness approaches, she is currently planning a mindfulness self-compassion course in Costa Rica, where 50% of the proceeds go to supporting Lands in Love, an animal shelter and community of plant-based animal lovers. Originally from Israel, Noah now lives in Los Angeles. Her current favourite art medium is paper cutouts, and she enjoys spending time with her spouse, children, and grandchildren.

References

Agren, T. (2014). Human reconsolidation: A reactivation and update. *Brain Research Bulletin, 105*, 70–82. https://doi.org/10.1016/j.brainresbull.2013.12.010

Barreiro, K. A., Suarez, L. D., Lynch, V. M., Molina, V. A., & Delorenzi, A. (2013). Memory expression is independent of memory labilization/reconsolidation. *Neurobiology of Learning and Memory, 106*, 283–291.

Baumeister, R. F., & Vohs, K. D. (2004). *Handbook of self-regulation.* Guilford Press.

Bremner, J. D. (2006). Stress and brain atrophy. *CNS Neurological Disorders Drug Targets, 5*(5), 503–512.

Brewin, C. R. (2018). Memory and forgetting. *Current Psychiatry Reports, 20*(87), 1–8. https://doi.org/10.1007/s11920-018-0950-7

Colcombe, S. J., Erickson, K. I., Raz, N., Webb, A. G., Cohen, N. J., McAuley, E., & Kramer, A. F. (2003). Aerobic fitness reduces brain tissue loss in aging humans. *Journal of Gerontology: Series A: Biological and Medical Sciences, 58*, M176–M180.

Collie, K., Backos, A., Malchiodi, C., & Spiegel, D. (2006). Art therapy for combat-related PTSD: Recommendations for research and practice. *Art Therapy: Journal of the American Art Therapy Association, 23*(4), 157–164.

De Gauna, M. I., Roibal, M. A., Ruiz, J. A., Fernández, J. I., & Bleichmar, H. B. (2015). Active change in psychodynamic therapy: Moments of high receptiveness. *American Journal of Psychotherapy, 69*(1), 65–86. https://doi: 10.1176/appi.psychotherapy.2015.69.1.65. PMID: 26241800

Ecker, B., Ticic, R., & Hulley, L. (2015). A primer on memory reconsolidation and its psychotherapeutic use as a core process of profound change. *The Neuropsychotherapist, 1*, 82–99. www.coherencetherapy.org/files/Ecker -etal-NPT2013April-Primer.pdf.

Elder, G. A., De Gasperi, R., & Gama Sosa, M. A. (2006). Research update: Neurogenesis in adult brain and neuropsychiatric disorders. *Mount Sinai Journal of Medicine, 73*(7), 931–940. Review.

Eriksson, P. S., Perfilieva, E., Bjork-Eriksson, T., Alborn, A. M., Nordborg, C., Peterson, D. A., & Gage, F. H. (1998). Neurogenesis in the adult human hippocampus. *Nature Medicine, 4*(11), 1313–1317.

Fougnie, D., & Marois, R. (2011, August 22). What limits working memory capacity? Evidence for modality-specific sources to the simultaneous storage of visual and auditory arrays. *Journal of Experimental Psychology: Learning, Memory, and Cognition*. Advance online publication. https://doi: 10.1037/a0024834

Fredrickson, B. L. (2013). Positive emotions broaden and build. In P. Devine & A. Plant (Eds.), *Advances in social psychology* (Vol. 47, pp. 1–53). Academic.

Gallese, V. (2003). The roots of empathy: The shared manifold hypothesis and the neural basis of intersubjectivity. *Psychopathology, 36*, 171–180.

Hartley, C. A., Gorun, A., Reddan, M. C., Ramirez, F., & Phelps, E. A. (2014). Stressor controllability modulates fear extinction in humans. *Neurobiology of Learning and Memory, 113*, 149–156. https://doi.org/10.1016/j.nlm.2013.12.003

Hass-Cohen, N. (2007). Cultural arts in action, musings on empathy. *GAINS Summer Quarterly*, 41–48.

Hass-Cohen, N. (2008). CREATE art therapy relational neuroscience principles (ATR-N). In N. Hass-Cohen & R. Carr (Eds.), *Art therapy and clinical neuroscience* (pp. 283–309). Jessica Kingsley Publishers.

Hass-Cohen, N. (2016). Secure resiliency: Art therapy relationship neuroscience trauma treatment principles and guidelines. In J. L. King (Ed.), *Art therapy, trauma and neuroscience: Theoretical and practical perspectives* (pp. 100–138). Routledge.

Hass-Cohen, N. (2018). Memory reconsolidation and art therapy-based conditions for prescriptive memory processes. In N. Gershman & B. E. Thompson (Eds.), *Grief therapy: Consolation through prescriptive memories*. Routledge.

Hass-Cohen, N., Bokoch, R., Clyde Findlay, J., & Banford Witting, A. (2018). A four-drawing art therapy trauma and resiliency protocol study. *The Arts in Psychotherapy, 61*, 44–56. https://doi.org/10.1016/j.aip.2018.02.003

Hass-Cohen, N., Bokoch, R., Goodman, K., & Conover, K. J. (2020). Pain drawing protocols: Quantitative results from a mixed method pilot study. *The Arts in Psychotherapy, 73*. https://doi.org/10.1016/j.aip.2020.101749

Hass-Cohen, N., & Carr, R. (Eds.). (2008). *Art therapy and clinial neuroscience*. Jessica Kingley Publisher.

Hass-Cohen, N., & Clyde Findlay, J. (2015). *Art therapy and the neuroscience of relationships, creativity, & resiliency skills and practices*. W. W. Norton.

Hass-Cohen, N., & Clyde Findlay, J. (2019). Memory reconsolidation in theory and practice: A proposed art therapy protocol. *The Arts in Psychotherapy, 63*, 51–59. https://doi.org/10.1016/j.aip.2019.03.002

Hass-Cohen, N., Clyde Findlay, J., Carr, R., & Vanderlan, J. (2014). "Check, change what you need to change and/or keep what you want": An art therapy neurobiological-based trauma protocol. *Art Therapy: Journal of the American Art Therapy Association, 31*(2), 69–78. https://doi.org/10.1080/07421656.2014.903825

Hull, A. (2002). Neuroimaging findings in post-traumatic stress disorder, systematic review. *British Journal of Psychiatry, 181*, 102–110.

Hupbach, A. (2011). The specific outcomes of reactivation-induced memory changes depend on the degree of competition between old and new information. *Frontiers in Behavioral Neuroscience, 5*(33), 1–2. https://doi.org/10.3389/fnbeh.2011.00033

Hupbach, A., Hardt, O., Gomez, O., & Nadel, L. (2008). The dynamics of memory. *Learning & Memory, 15*, 574–579.

Jennings, S. (2011). *Healthy attachments and neuro-dramatic-play*. Jessica Kingsley Publishers.

Kravits, K. (2008). The stress response and adaptation theory. In N. Hass-Cohen & R. Carr (Eds.), *Art therapy and clinical neuroscience*. Jessica Kingsley Publishers.

Lane, R. D., Ryan, L., Nadel, L., & Greenberg, L. (2015). Memory reconsolidation, emotional arousal, and the process of change in psychotherapy: New insights from brain science. *The Behavioral and Brain Sciences*. https://.doi.org/10.1017/S0140525X14000041 (Published online. 19 pages).

Lazar, S. W., Kerrb, C. E., Wasserman, R. H., Gray, J. R., Greved, D. N., Treadwaya, M. T., McGarvey, M., Quinn, B. T., Dusek, J. A., Benson, H., Rauch, S. L., Moore, C. I., & Fischl, B. (2005). Meditation experience is associated with increased cortical thickness. *Neuroreport, 16*(17), 1893–1897.

LeDoux, J. E. (2000). Emotion circuits in the brain. *Annual Review of Neuroscience, 23*, 155–184. https://doi:10.1146/annurev.neuro.23.1.155

Lee, J. L. C., Nader, K., & Schiller, D. (2017). An update on memory reconsolidation updating. *Trends in Cognitive Science, 21*(7), 531–545. https://doi.org/10.1016/j.tics 2017.04.006

Luck, S. J., & Vogel, E. K. (2013). Visual working memory capacity: From psychophysics and neurobiology to individual differences. *Trends in Cognitive Science, 17*(8), 391–400. https://doi.org/10.1016/j.tics.2013.06.006 (review)

McEwen, B., & Lasley, E. N. (2002). *The end of stress as we know it*. National Academies Press.

McNamee, C. M. (2003). Bilateral art: Facilitating systemic integration and balance. *The Arts in Psychotherapy, 30*, 283–292.

Murphy, S. E., Clare, M., O'Donoghue, E., Drazich, S. H., Blackwell, S. E., Nobre, A. E., & Holmes, E. A (2015). Imagining a brighter future: The effect of positive imagery training on mood, prospective mental imagery and emotional bias in older adults. *Psychiatry Research, 230*(1), 36–43.

Nader, K., Schafe, G. E., & LeDoux, J. E. (2000). The labile nature of consolidation theory. *Biological Psychiatry 15, 76*(4), 274–280.

Porges, S. W. (2001). The polyvagal theory: Phylogenetic substrates of a social nervous system. *International Journal of Psychophysiology, 42*, 123–146.

Porges, S. W., Bazhenova, O. V., Bal, E., Carlson, N., Sorokin, Y., Heilman, K. J., Cook, E. H., & Lewis, G. F. (2014). Reducing hypersensitivities in autistic spectrum disorder: Preliminary findings evaluating the listening project protocol (A precursor to the safe and sound protocol). *Frontiers in Pediatrics, 2*, 80.

Prasko, J., Horacek, J., Zalesky, R., Kopecek, M., Novak, T., Paskova, B., Skrdlantova, L., Belohlavek, O., & Hoschl, C. (2004). The change of regional brain metabolism (18FDG PET) in panic disorder during the treatment with cognitive behavioral therapy or antidepressants. *Neuroendocrinology Letters, 25*(5), 340–348. *Relationships, creativity, and resiliency: Skills and practices*. W. W. Norton.

Schiller, D., Monfils, M. H., Raio, C. M., Johnson, D. C., Ledoux, J. E., & Phelps, E. A. (2010). Preventing the return of fear in humans using reconsolidation update mechanisms. *Nature, 7*(7277), 49–53.

Schore, A. (2007, February 2, 3). *The science of the art of psychotherapy* [conference]. Skirball Cultural Center, Los Angeles, CA.

Schwabe, L., Nader, K., & Pruessner, J. C. (2014). Reconsolidation of human memory: Brain mechanisms and clinical relevance. *Biological Psychiatry, 76*(4), 274–280.

Silva, M. B., & Soares, A. B. (2018). Reconsolidation of human motor memory: From boundary conditions to behavioral interventions-how far are we from clinical applications? *Behavioral Brain Research, 353*, 83–90. https://doi: 10.1016/j.bbr.2018.07.003. Epub 2018 Jul 3. PMID: 29983391

Simon, K. C., Nadel, L., & Gómez, R. L. (2020). Parameters of memory reconsolidation: Learning mode influences likelihood of memory modification. *Frontiers in Behavioral Neuroscience, 14*, 120. https://doi: 10.3389/fnbeh.2020.00120. PMID: 33192353; PMCID: PMC7542095

Straube, T., Glauer, M., Dilger, S., Mentzel, H. J., & Miltner, W. H. (2006). Effects of cognitive-behavioral therapy on brain activation in specific phobia. *Neuroimage, 29*(1), 125–135.

Taylor, S. E. (2006). Tend and befriend biobehavioral bases of affiliation under stress. *Current Directions in Psychological Science, 5*(6), 273–277. doi:10.1111/j.1467-8721.2006.00451

Tronson, N. C., & Taylor, J. R. (2007). Molecular mechanisms of memory reconsolidation. *Nature Reviews Neuroscience, 8*, 262–275. https://doi.org/10.1038/nrn2090

Wichert, S., Wolf, O. T., & Schwabe, L. (2013). Updating of episodic memories depends on the strength of new learning after memory reconsolidation. *Behavioral Neuroscience, 127*(3), 331–338. https://doi.org/10.1037/a0032028

Part I

Setting the scene

Arts therapists writing a book in the time of COVID-19 pandemic

A compilation of personal reactions arranged by major themes

Alison Talmage, Agnès Desombiaux-Sigley, Caroline Miller, Daphne Rickson, Kim Hau Pang, Mariana Torkington, Pamela Dunne, Renda Dionne Madrigal, Sarah Mann Shaw, Sian Palmer, Vanitha Chandrasegaram, and Verity Danbold

Writing a book in 2020–21, with an international cast of twelve writers, many of the ordinary misfortunes of life befell the writers. One had a broken wrist; another, a broken leg; others, bronchitis, death of family members, bushfires and floods, moving house (three writers), moving cities, moving countries, setting up a trust, catching COVID-19; four emergency hospitalisations for other events; and continuing to work hard, take on new ideas, and collaborate with colleagues. Then came a pandemic, and COVID-19 entered all our vocabularies and our lives and relationships.

Personal stressors and disasters continued as usual, overlaid with lockdowns, changing government edicts, changing governments. There was no uniform international response, with governments showing different levels of respect and relationship with the populace. Some sought to strengthen dictatorial inclinations; others used new legislation to change our behaviour and try to control the spread of disease; still others tried persuasion and inclusion and increased communication to try to gain the support of the largest part of the population. Numbers of people, already suspicious of government, were drawn into increasingly complex conspiracy theories which gave them a rationale for dismissing the whole COVID-19 crisis. Some engaged in increased religious behaviour; others in increased spiritual self-examination in relation to death and the meaning and purpose of our continuing lives.

Themes from individual group member responses to the impact of COVID-19

Work

In the years of COVID-19 we have all had to change our practice, often to working remotely and connecting electronically with clients. Generally, change has led to reflection about the essentials of our practice and how to retain these.

DOI: 10.4324/9781003082897-2

Often there has been a greater demand from our clients which has challenged our ways of working and led to new approaches. Of course, some arts therapists also lost jobs and had to find ways to create new work.

Working online, virtually, was manageable in the short term but continuing in the longer term raised questions about essential elements of relationship and when working with transference and the body.

Before the pandemic, when dramatherapy groups were generally held in person, some dramatherapists used a combination of in person and Zoom. The Zoom participants were treated the same way as in-person participants and always participated in the enactments, movement, or creative arts activities. They were able to share art, photos, video, and written work through the shared screen function. The switch to Zoom only was not a big adjustment, but it did require greater creativity in how to use it with more breakout rooms, and the whiteboard, and turning the video on and off in games. The ethical issues of using Zoom in disclosure statements, which participants signed, had to be addressed along with what now constituted safe practice. Some physical safety issues were approached with the use of blue filters on glasses. Young children were more difficult to engage on Zoom, even with the most creative of activities. There were some benefits during the pandemic as participants had more time for classes and therapy, but others wanted to see the therapist in person and did not accept remote contact.

With national and regional lockdowns in each country, some therapists moved all their practices online, including offering online training. In turn, this meant redesigning consents and contracts. There was often a need for therapists to engage in further training about how to work creatively online. One therapist noticed how the dissonance of working online seemed to make the brain work harder, leading to earlier exhaustion. Wanting to continue to offer a containing and creative space for clients, some were delighted to find new ways of creating images and stories, of doing puppet play, mirroring and movement, and role-play.

There was a reported sense of relief when able to offer some face-to-face sessions in COVID-secure physical environments. The clients who were most glad to be back were adolescents and young adults. They seemed to really appreciate, and need, the embodied physical presence of the therapist. This also felt easier for many therapists. However, other extremely anxious and/or autistic clients continued to find working online more helpful.

> Pandemic lockdowns might be pervasive, but not all our movements are restricted. This has led to a rise in dance, as people seek fitness, stress relief, healing – and connection. Live classes on Instagram and YouTube have proliferated.
>
> (Malozzi, 2020)

Some online art and art therapy programmes have been developed to allow people to use art in an intentional way while in isolation. In other situations, individuals have offered their own art on various internet platforms to stimulate interaction with others around the artworks.

In some situations, healthcare workers were required to be tested on a regular basis. Inpatient and day-care services were separated, which affected the spaces which could be used for therapy. There were restrictions on social and group-based activities for inpatients. Increased liaisons between some music therapists, art therapists, and physical and occupational therapists, enabled them to devise creative approaches.

Online practice widened dancing circles across the globe. Dance can connect us with our common humanity, unique creativity, and capacity to co-create the best possible future. We witnessed moments of deep resonance and generativity between and among dancers: hand gestures of giving and taking, mirroring movements that spoke of seeing and being seen, dancers moving with emotion and feeling supported. Ripples of rhythm and patterns of movement in the whole group came from the dance floor at home. We are the circle, the circle is us. Moving in circle accessed our natural orientation towards safety, connection, and collaboration, creating a feeling of wholeness, interdependence, and well-being. Online group members have reflected that they felt deeply connected to themselves, to one another and to their families, and even to their ancestors.

Music therapists in New Zealand created a tile collage of their photos and a verbal collage of their COVID-19 personal and professional actions and reactions in a large-scale collaborative article for their professional journal. They pointed to virtual choirs and livestreamed music, with an increase in music for well-being available on the internet. They also highlighted the importance of all arts therapists continuing to write of our personal and professional experiences, including our continuing research, for the ongoing professional development of all members and of our professions.

The environment and community

For many, the threat of COVID-19 underlined the necessity of looking after the environment and building strong communities, a sense that 'we are all in this together'. Perhaps there was an acceleration of the urgency to change the way we live together, to realise how every action, every decision we take can affect the planet and others. It reinforced the idea of our interdependency and need for common goals. While there was an inundation of plastic, there was less environmental pollution from traffic, more bird song, and more peaceful sound environments with reduced traffic and industrial noise. Daily newspapers and television stressed the importance of the health of the community. Physical health concerns often led to more thought for neighbours and neighbourhoods. People worked together to support those who were isolated, ill, or unable to provide necessities, such as food or company, through periods of the lockdown or other restricted movement. Some supported organisations providing food, as the growing crisis amplified social, economic, and health disparities experienced by disenfranchised peoples across the globe. Focus on the crisis response in the United States brought 'black lives matter' into international concern as the realities of inequity in global social systems throughout the world became apparent. This highlighted similar inequities in many countries and how our local practice might disadvantage a range of ethnic and national groups. It became evident that the communities already under social and economic stress often suffered the worst consequences of COVID-19 responses. It then appeared that many of those communities would also have poorer access to vaccinations.

Personal/emotional changes

Some governments have shown a lot of strength, determination, direction, care, genuineness, and decency and worked closely with public health experts to make informed decisions in an unknown territory. Some citizens felt safe, protected, and reassured that the crisis was managed as well as could be. In other countries, a lack of confidence in the handling of the pandemic lead to societal and political divisions. These had a further impact on personal health.

Clients presented with anxiety, depression, existential fears, worries about conspiracy theories, and daily stresses of broken relationships, losing jobs, family strife and violence, and huge amounts of uncertainty and anxiety. Therapists also experienced all of these and had to call on a wide range of personal resources to keep focused on clients. Therapists found their own resilience in creativity and solidarity and new learning, amidst uncertainty about how long they might be planning for. Self-care as a therapist has become even more significant.

During the COVID-19 pandemic, we witnessed and experienced fear, uncertainty, and isolation. Dancing in and holding online classes demonstrated how dancing offers both remedy and prevention. Dance calms our nervous systems, lifts our spirits, and maintains our connections with each other. In working online with dancers practising on their own at home, it was important to create the necessary conditions and facilitate in ways that supported connection. Many felt lonely and isolated during the lockdown, missing physical touch and the feeling of dancing together in community. "More than ever, we need to dance with purpose to remind the world that humanity still exists", says Gregory Vuyani Maqoma, an acclaimed dancer and educator from South Africa. "Our purpose is one that strives to change the world one step at a time" (Malozzi, 2020).

Behavioural changes

Mask wearing, contact tracing, and lockdowns brought new vocabulary as well as new behaviour. There was new learning about legal issues in this new context. Students in training missed opportunities to work with clients and had to grapple with online courses, newly devised by their lecturers. Programmes had to be rewritten. Days took on a different shape with new patterns and activities of self-care, meditation, relaxation, and exercise. Professional liaisons became focused on technological matters more than client problems in some instances. The internet became a source for bringing creativity into technological therapeutic encounters, and distant contact with colleagues exchanging ideas. For many people art, music, drama, and dance continued to be important and became important in other ways. Finding connection with other people through these continued.

Writing this book

The focus for this book was already on how the arts therapies are adapted in different countries and with different populations of clients and on the way our practice is becoming informed by research from neuroscience. In focusing on the findings from neuroscience, we have found additional support for our ways of working with the arts therapies. None of this changes the essential nature of our practice of developing relationship, attending closely to the client, and supporting the client to become the change agent for their own lives. We are still relational beings who must find ways to stay connected in specific and appropriate ways. We connect with others through our skin, senses, and the whole of our central and peripheral nervous systems. The pandemic has helped us relearn the importance of this connection and to find new ways to connect.

Further reading

Cluloo, M. B. C. (2020). Afterword. *New Zealand Journal of Music Therapy, 18*, 7–66. www.musictherapy.org.nz/journal/2020-2/

Gipson, L. R., Williams, B., & Norris, M. (2020). Commentary. Three black women's reflections on Covid-19 and creative arts therapies then and now. *Voices, 20*(2). doi:10.15845/*voices*.v2012.3115

Hill, M. A. (2020). Drama therapy during Covid-19: A digital call to adventure. *Polyphony Journal of the Irish Association of Creative Arts Therapists*. https:// polyphony.iacat.me/drama-therapy-during-covid-19-a-call-to-digital-adventure

Malozzi, M. (2020). Virtual dance parties. What's behind their rise? *National Geographic* www.nationalgeographic.com/travel/2020/04/how-dance-connects-people-during-coronavirus/

Talmage, A., & Clulee, M. B. C. (2020). Fostering creativity and collaboration [Editorial]. *New Zealand Journal of Music Therapy, 18*, 1–6.

Talmage, A., Clulee, M. B. C., Cho, H., Glass, M., Gordon, J. S., Kong, J. C., Hoskyns, S., Hunt, E. L., Hunt, B. J., Jeong, A. A. Y., Johns, L., Matthews, E., Rickson, D., Riegelhaupt Landreani, C., Sabri, S., & Solly, R. (2020). Music therapy in time of pandemic: Experiences of telehealth, self-care, and resource oriented practice during Covid-19 in New Zealand. *New Zealand Journal of Music Therapy, 18*, 7–66. www.musictherapy.org.nz/journal/2020-2/

Introduction

Caroline Miller

Neuroscience continues to uncover new connections with, and between, the arts therapies which both confirm current ways of working as arts therapists and suggest new ones. The arts therapies make specific calls which stimulate creativity, with creativity seen as a major healing agent. They do this with creative methods and materials and through the physicality of the arts therapies which stimulate embodiment and integration of new learning. The embodiment, creativity, and interaction which are part of dramatherapy, dance/movement therapy, music therapy, and art therapy all have direct links with the human nervous system through several routes. This can lead to a productive interaction between the arts therapies and neuroscience in which arts therapists begin to link the work of, and with, the client to its impact on the nervous system and even begin to plan therapy to stimulate and develop specific parts of the nervous system to tap into the brain plasticity now known to exist throughout the life span. Each chapter in this book relates work with specific clients or client groups, in particular countries and cultural settings, and with links to relevant neuroscience.

The writers work in the following countries: South Africa, New Zealand (NZ), the UK, the US, Malaysia, and Singapore. One from Australia works in the UK and has worked in India, giving her a perspective on the importance of access to movement-based therapy across countries and cultures. Of the four NZ writers, three have migrated to NZ from the UK, France, and South American countries. They bring their own cultural backgrounds and the experience of migration to their work. Two of their chapters are accounts of work with their clients who also migrated to NZ. The South African writes of an occasion when ancient dance tradition brought together a large group of women representing the diverse countries and languages of the African continent.

Some of the writers trained outside of their own countries of origin and then became pioneers in finding a path to working with specific cultures within their home countries. Four of the writers have English as their second language. Even the first-language English speakers returned home with the new language of the arts therapies and had to undertake the task of fitting the

DOI: 10.4324/9781003082897-3

training and therapeutic culture into their local country and culture. Most of the countries represented by the writers of this book have initiated their own local training programmes, with associated professional bodies and professional journals. However, the wider (English-speaking European world) seldom hears of the creative therapy work being done outside of Europe, the UK, and the US. This book begins to bring those voices less heard. The writers use case study and recent research material to illustrate the latest advances in the practice of the arts therapies in New Zealand, South-East Asia, South Africa, the US, and the UK. In each chapter, client names are changed to protect their privacy.

This book uses case study and recent research material to illustrate the latest advances in the practice of the arts therapies. It outlines specific properties of arts therapies approaches which link to findings about neurological changes through therapy. The various chapters illustrate work with children with experience of autism or experience of trauma, with groups of adults and groups of adolescents, and with adults with neurological disorders.

Summary of chapters

Chapter 1. Arts therapies: recent advances

Caroline Miller

The relationship of the arts therapies to humanistic and psychodynamic approaches to therapy and counselling is considered along with a relatively new understanding of brain plasticity and many other findings from neuroscience. We can see that all therapeutic approaches can enhance neurological and behavioural changes. This chapter introduces specific ways in which the arts therapies may do that. This includes the role of creativity and the engagement of body and mind in neurologically enhancing therapeutic effects. These are further illustrated in the subsequent chapters.

Chapter 2. Exploring implicit memory through metaphor: Jonah and the missing heart; a story of attachment and dramatherapy

Sarah Mann Shaw

Sarah Mann Shaw works with adopted children in the United Kingdom. Her clients have experienced trauma and loss at early ages when they have been unable to develop a coherent system of making meaning around these experiences. Sarah works within a framework of implicit and explicit memory to help children form a coherent understanding of their past and present experiences. This leads to an understanding of the impact of current experiences which elicit physical and emotional reactions triggered from past experiences.

Sarah works with dramatherapy and metaphor to enable her clients to live in the present without being overwhelmed by experiences from the past. Dramatherapists refer to this as aesthetic distance.

Sarah's account is of a young child who had experienced trauma and neglect. She joined in his play with puppets, toys, and metaphor as a co-creator of a new understanding of his life in his adoptive family. Sarah's work was warm, rich, and communicative while she kept track of the neurological development and the emotional repair he needed. She worked with this child in the presence of his adoptive mother, who was able to find a new appreciation of him and to find new ways of interacting with him to strengthen their attachment bonds.

Sarah tracked change with this client by using part of PSYCHLOPS to help him identify the immediate problem, through the framework of Sue Jennings Neurodevelopmental Play model (2011), and by using an immediate overt reflecting model within sessions to articulate and name his metaphorical and developmental work.

Chapter 3. Narradrama as a Three Act Play: transformation, neurobiology, and discovery

Pamela Dunne and Renda Dionne Madrigal

Narradrama as a Three Act Play (NTAP) is a subset of Narradrama, which is the integration of dramatherapy, narrative, and the creative arts. This chapter details the tenets of this therapeutic process, which include the development of a creative, individual script by each participant that explores personal issues through the creation of preferred roles, alternative stories, and preferred outcomes. NTAP offers a unique approach to the writing, development, and performance of a play while offering expanded opportunities for self-growth through integration of personalised exercises.

Narradrama is influenced by positive psychology and narrative therapy. It is grounded in a humanistic belief that we all possess propensity for positive change and agency in our own healing. It also incorporates principles and research from interpersonal neurobiology and the study of positive emotions. NTAP is a group process and therefore inherently connects individuals to one another. NTAP also creates an additional value due to its collaborative, supportive, creative, and therapeutic process.

The writers used community-based participatory research, narrative research, and practice-based research as theoretical frameworks for evaluating this work. It was experimental in three ways – NTAP developed from Narradrama, the population worked with, and working with Zoom technology.

Chapter 4. Dramatherapy with adolescents in Malaysia: Be

Vanitha Chandrasegaram

Vanitha Chandrasegaram, in Malaysia, reflects on work she did with a group of drama students at an international school. The students participated in six dramatherapy sessions which allowed them to develop group relationships, spontaneity, and gradual intimacy around issues relating to their age group and gender. They found many commonalities, although they came from different countries and diverse cultural and ethnic groups.

The group members were all young women who were working together in a drama class to create a short play to perform to an audience as part of a final assessment in drama. The dramatherapy sessions provided additional opportunities to strengthen interpersonal bonds as well as personal confidence and the opportunity to reflect and to share reflections. Within the dramatherapy sessions, themes were identified which became the core of the final performance piece. Vanitha writes with an awareness of the relevant and significant neuroscience findings underlying the development of trusting and supportive relationships in dramatherapy groups.

The main identified changes were increased trust, mutual support, and openness among group members, which were reported through feedback from the group and individuals, from their confidence in the final performance, and from feedback from the audience members at that performance.

Chapter 5. A multi-theoretical, multimodal, arts–psychotherapy approach to trauma and depression

Agnès Desombiaux-Sigley

Agnès Desombiaux-Sigley was educated in France and now lives in NZ. She reflects on work with a client, with a similar background in France, who also migrated to NZ. Her client wanted to work with a therapist of similar cultural background and language as she explored her family issues of depression, loss, trauma, and grief.

Working with many traumatised clients led Agnès to further training in somatic therapy with clients with trauma. As she developed greater awareness of how embodied her clients' experiences were, she developed awareness of physical reactions she experienced in response to them. She reflects on these as mirrors to the clients' psychic and somatic experiences in the present in therapy which resonated within her own physical body. For this chapter, Agnès took a new view on her work with this client by focusing on her own somatic countertransference while working with this client. She reviewed the client's artwork through the lens of counter-transferential somatic response, tracking changes for the client in conjunction with her therapy notes from the time.

Agnès's work is supported by the work of Merleau-Ponty on the phenomenology of perception and the polyvagal theory of Porges and Schore, among many others, as she weaves attachment theory, loss and grief, and childhood trauma within her integrative arts therapies approach.

Chapter 6. *We are here together for a while: art therapy initiatives within a hospice setting in Singapore*

Kim Hau Pang

Pang's work shows art therapy as a community resource in the hands of a resourceful therapist. His work demonstrates how art therapy can be contextualised for different population groups and their needs, even within a single setting. He and his art therapist colleague arrange individual sessions for clients and families in hospice care. Additionally, using the Men's Shed model, he arranged for a facilitated space to be provided within the hospice day-care centre, where men could gather to make things and, in doing so, to form a supportive community. One of the regular participants named the group Men United.

Kim Hau Pang includes co-facilitation with colleagues, as well as providing them with art spaces to work, alone or together, to process some of their work with clients, or to support their own resilience in the face of grief and loss. He is part of a group which brings families of all faiths together at biennial church services during which they collectively remember their family members who have passed through hospice care. This is a community-oriented initiative through which people can also participate through the arts.

Each initiative centres on the universality of grief and loss as a human experience within the hospice model of living the best life possible right up to death.

Pang tracks change through ecological methods like asking the men in the Men's Shed to provide qualitative accounts, by his own observation of mood and behaviour changes over time, and through attendance and participation in supportive staff activities including the Interfaith gathering.

Chapter 7. *Imagination and art therapy: a bridge to transformation for traumatised clients*

Mariana Torkington

Mariana explores the role of imagination in the treatment of trauma. She provides an example from her work with a child immigrant from an African country now living in NZ. The child 'Flora', worked with Mariana for 18 months, and then returned for a review three years after therapy had ended. In that review Mariana was able to reflect, with Flora, on the artwork done during therapy. In a further reflective review, Mariana used the CREATE neuro-relational model of Hass-Cohen and Findlay, alongside a psychodynamic model of de Rivera, as lenses to examine the changes Flora made during therapy. Mariana's practice of art therapy is informed by principles of Jungian psychology, psychodynamic psychotherapy, and humanistic psychology, acknowledging the place of spirituality as an integral part of the psyche. Research into neuroscience and neuroplasticity provided a new lens for Mariana to further examine the importance of imagination as a necessary component of change.

Chapter 8. Singing all together in the CeleBRation choir: a music therapist's perspective on community singing for adults who have neurogenic communication difficulties

Alison Talmage

Alison writes of her ongoing research with singing groups for adults with acquired neurological disorders, including stroke, Parkinson's disease, and the dementias, and their associated communication difficulties. She works in the context of singing for well-being, with music therapy and interdisciplinary approaches within a biopsychosocial–spiritual framework. This is a specific context within the broader field of singing-focused music therapy. Choir membership is a strengths-based response to social isolation and quality-of-life (QoL) needs, and the author is involved in QoL research with the choir. Shared singing is studied as speech–language–voice maintenance/rehabilitation in this group. Questions which arise include, what is practical, meaningful, and measurable in practice, as well as in research? Vignettes might include poetry and original song lyrics written by choir members. After considering several possibilities, Alison opted for action research methods as the most suitable for this kind of study.

Chapter 9. Music therapy for autistic children: responding to contemporary understandings with new research approaches

Daphne Rickson

Daphne Rickson recognises the multitude of personal characteristics and abilities of autistic children which often include musical interests and abilities. This means that music can become a major source of pleasure, engagement, and a means of communication and relationship. Using musical contact as an alternative to the more difficult linguistic and social norms and methods can ease an entry into those more standardised social forms of relationship and communication. Daphne describes autism as a disability rather than a disorder, reflecting its place within human variability. Music can provide a means of communication through which autistic children improve executive functioning in the brain.

Daphne describes 'a multiple mixed-methods case study design to investigate the perceived impact of music therapy in supporting the interpersonal communication of autistic children and their social skill development across a series of sessions of music therapy. Learning stories, video, descriptions of sessions, and photographs contributed material which was collected to be examined by teams of evaluators.

Chapter 10. In circle: the benefits of dance as a community practice

Sian Palmer

Sian Palmer reflects on a conference (African Women in Dialogue, AFWID) in Johannesburg, where she led a group of women in expressive movement. The women, who represented numerous African countries and a multitude of different languages, spiritual beliefs, and cultural practices, found common ground in dancing and stamping in circles. Sian links these dance and movement traditions to the cultural practices of ancient African peoples near the cradle of humanity. The offering spoke to the feminine African way – being rooted in the body and shared in circle. The focus was on the theme of 'journeys' – sharing stories of surviving and thriving. Sian reviews these practices and occasions with new understanding from neuroscience about relationship building and connecting through joint activity grounded in ancient tradition. Sian was born in Johannesburg and says that, as a white South African–born and European-trained therapist, she is of both the South and the North. She created expressive movement because of her trust in embodied creative expression and her practice as a Sesame therapist. The Sesame approach was created after Marion Lindkvist spent time with traditional healers in South Africa.

This chapter demonstrates body-based therapy, bringing together a disparate group with common traditions communicating, joining, and connecting through movement. Sian observed the changes in posture and action from isolation and withdrawal to warm and vivid communication. She had a later opportunity to receive feedback from a conference participant, whose observations of how the circle dancing had brought participants closer together supported her own observations and records from the conference event.

Chapter 11. Mind and movement: using the universality of neuroscience in dance movement therapy

Verity Danbold

Verity explores ways that neuroscience can help to lead us to a more global approach to therapy. While many existing therapies may be Eurocentric in their approach with a strong emphasis on the individual self and strict boundaries of time and length of therapy, grounding it in neuroscience encourages therapeutic approaches to come from a more universal base: the brain and the body working together. Dance movement therapy furthers this by working through the body, allowing for non-verbal intervention, and recognising that all movement is valid. Breathwork can form a universal base as breathing is something that we all do regardless of culture, age, and gender.

Verity's writing expands our views to consider more global perspectives including matters of equity, resource use, and political considerations, as issues of relevance to us all wherever we work and whatever our training.

Considerations of outcomes and research

Arts therapists are increasingly aware of the need to be able to report outcomes of therapy in a comprehensible way, indicating what change means and how change is noted. This adds an additional level of understanding about the effects of therapy, for therapists, and for clients and their families, as well as for colleagues of other disciplines.

There are modality specific measures which arts therapists have used alongside standardised measures developed and used by public health specialists, psychologists, or other mental health workers. These chapters show an array of measures used in a variety of settings for a variety of purposes. Daphne Rickson, Pamela Dunne, and Renda Dionne Madrigal are all engaged in ongoing research and in teaching others. Alison Talmage uses the QoL measure developed for large public health populations and widely used in public health settings. Daphne Rickson continues a quest to find client friendly ways to measure the effect of music therapy on the communications of young people with autism. Pamela Dunne and Renda Dionne Madrigal have engaged with ecologically based research methods and used a combination of practice-based research and community-based research for their groundbreaking work with a small group of Native Americans and black Americans. Kim Hau Pang and his colleagues have widened community involvement in aspects of hospice care, in which they use qualitative and ecological approaches to gauge changes in individual and community responses to their programmes.

In Malaysia, Vanitha Chandrasegaram involved group members in discussion and feedback and monitored increased engagement in group relationships and creativity. The final performance was followed by audience and participant feedback, and with qualitative feedback from the participants as an ongoing part of the group process. Sian Palmer brought dance to a large, diverse group of African women at a conference. She utilised observation, reflective practice, and participant feedback to gauge the impact of the large group session.

Sarah Mann Shaw tracked behavioural and neurological changes, with inferences about the connections between the two, in a deliberate sequencing of play events designed to develop explicit memories making sense to the client from his implicit memories which could not be named or related in any coherent way. Sarah used an ongoing reflexive process with her child client and used Jenning's model of neurodramatic play as both an assessment frame and a guide to continuing therapeutic work. She also referred to elements of PSYCHLOPS (an assessment for children) as part of helping the child to identify a central problem.

Agnès Desombiaux-Sigley worked within a frame of transference and embodied countertransference. She used a reflective process in retrospectively reviewing her client's artwork and past and post–therapy review responses. This followed a qualitative, autoethnographic process.

Mariana Torkington's client completed a CORS (Child Outcome Rating Scale), a self-assessment questionnaire, which allowed a comparison of her ratings across a range of settings before and after her series of therapy sessions.

Verity Danbold, taking a global view of mental health provision, utilises official publications of agencies like World Health Organization and United Nations Educational, Scientific and Cultural Organisation, and their stated aims. She critiques practice in the light of stated policy for a high standard of mental health care and general health care, which should be universally available but which generally is not. She advocates for wider access to dance movement therapy as a low-cost and effective resource to meet some of these officially identified needs.

References/Further reading

Cornwall, A., & Jewkes, R. (1995). What is participatory research? *Social Science & Medicine, 41*, 1667–1676.

de Rivera, J. L. G. (1992). *The stages of psychotherapy. European Journal of Psychiatry, 6*(1), 51–58.

Hass-Cohen, N., & Findlay, J. C. (2015). *Art therapy and the neuroscience of relationships, creativity and resiliency skills and practices.* W. W. Norton.

Haythorne, D., Crockford, S., & Godfrey, E. (2012). Roundabout and the development of PSYCHLOPS kids evaluation, Chp. 18. In L. Leigh, I. Gersch, A. Dix, & D. Haythorne (Eds.), *Dramatherapy with children, young people and schools: Enabling creativity, sociability, communication and learning.* Routledge.

Jenkins, B., Storie, S., & Purdy, S. C. (2017). Quality of life for individuals with a neurological condition who participate in social/therapeutic choirs. *New Zealand Journal of Music Therapy, 15*, 59–94.

Jennings, S. (2011). *Healthy attachment and neurodevelopmental play.* Jessica Kingsley Publishers.

Merleau-Ponty, M. (1962). *The phenomenology of perception.* Routledge and Kegan Paul.

Miller, C. (2017). Practice-based evidence: Therapist as researcher, using outcome measures. *Dramatherapy, 38*(1), 4–15.

Miller, S. D., Duncan, B. L., Brown, J., Sparks, J. A., & Claud, D. A. (2003). The outcome rating scale: A preliminary study of the reliability, validity and feasibility of a brief visual analog measure. *Journal of Brief Therapy, 2*(2), 91–100.

Moen, T. (2006). Reflections on the narrative research approach. *International Journal of Qualitative Methodology, 5*(4), 1–10.

Porges, S. W. (2011). *The polyvagal theory: Neurophysiological foundations of emotions, attachment, communication, and self-regulation.* W. W. Norton.

Redstone, A. (2004). Researching people's experience of narrative therapy: Acknowledging the contribution of the client to what works in counselling conversations. *International Journal of Narrative Therapy and Community Work, 2*, 1–6.

Schore, A. N. (2019). *Right brain psychotherapy.* Norton Professional Books.

Soth, M. (2018). *Embodied countertransference.* www.researchgate.net/publication/322918578 _Embodied_Countertransference

Tootell, A. (2004). Decentering research practice. *International Journal of Narrative Therapy and Community Work, 3,* 54–66.

1 Arts therapies

Recent advances

Caroline Miller

Arts therapies and neuroscience

The arts therapies are aligned with humanistic, psychodynamic, narrative, and other theoretical approaches, with specific characteristics related to the arts and creativity. Most therapies seek to find the creative impulse in clients, as this is a dynamic factor in identifying areas of desired change, and then the personal resources that might enable that change. Key to successful therapy and therapeutic engagement and outcome is the therapeutic relationship where clients feel that they are in a safe environment. Arts therapists work to stimulate creativity and to build a safe and cooperative environment using creative methods and materials to stimulate engagement and develop a relationship. In addition, art, music, drama, and dance/movement therapies work in an embodied way with physical action working directly with the brain and nervous system. This means they are particularly well suited to working with attachment issues and those related to trauma, as well as other common issues that clients present.

Pitruzzella (2009) writes of creativity as a "hidden connecting principle". He describes the games and warm-ups of dramatherapy as a "play of encounter". He sees creativity as including curiosity, versatility, and presence, which affect how we encounter the world and give experiences meaning. In improvisation, we respond in the moment experimenting with each other, and in planning for group enactments, we develop trust and reciprocity. This reflects Siegel's (2012) work on interpersonal neurobiology. Dunne (2017) describes dramatherapy as strengthening neural networks and brain plasticity through embodiment, repetition, dramatic projection, new experiences, positive emotional arousal, and distancing among other benefits. Csikszentmihalyi (1996) introduced the idea of flow as the basis of creativity, and arts therapists use materials and techniques to induce such a state. The arts therapies use art, music, drama, and dance/ movement, sometimes in combination, as the third element in therapy along with therapist and client, as they focus on relationship building and safety in the relationship and in the therapeutic setting.

The arts have a long history in every society. They are used, in cave art and subsequent arts forms, to record the daily activities of communities and the practices of importance to them. They hold the stories, beliefs, and histories of groups.

DOI: 10.4324/9781003082897-4

They are used with the intent to heal and for entertainment, for developing community solidarity, for reflecting the beliefs of communities, and for teaching the history, beliefs, and rituals that mark significant life stages. The arts therapies have developed from these traditions. During the past century, the arts therapies have become more prominent in offering psychological therapies. They have found common ground along with humanistic and psychodynamic theoretical approaches to therapy and counselling, with relatively new understanding of brain plasticity. We can see that all therapeutic approaches can enhance neurological and behavioural changes. This book looks at specific ways in which the arts therapies do that. Many of these are sensory and relational; some are inherently developmental. As examples, music may use rhythm and communicate through changing rhythms or playing musical instruments, with non-verbal communication or with joint playing and singing enhancing group connectedness. McGrath (2017) writes:

> Where adverse life events negatively impact on the ability to regulate both physiologically and emotionally, therapeutic interventions that are grounded in music and rhythm can support and enhance the growth, integration and repair of the self.

Art uses a variety of media with hands directly interacting with media or using tools like brushes or palette knives, as well as stimulating the senses with a range of colours. Dramatherapy uses physical activities to warm up the whole body and mind and the connection with others in group work, as well as through interesting props, costumes, stories, and acting out stories or scenes. Dance movement therapy (DMT) similarly uses the body, with connection through gross to subtle movement and expression and communication and control. All contain an element of play, with storytelling, communication, drama, and sensory involvement. Malchiodi (2014) argues that these activities facilitate a creative sense of self-exploration that connects mind and body stimulating each of the senses. She considers that they have an important relationship with neuroscience because they emphasise

(a) "sensory based interventions
(b) nonverbal communication
(c) right hemisphere dominance
(d) emotional regulation
(e) relational strategies
(f) arts therapies can be used with children, adolescents, and adults".

(Kottman et al., 2017, p. 51)

Neuroscience adds to the established practices of the arts therapies by

1 providing a rationale for specific practices and approaches,
2 offering the possibility of targeting therapy to specific brain areas,

3   giving a rationale for behaviours and reactions observed,
4   clarifying functions of different brain areas and optimal interactions between these,
5   outlining a map of brain development, and
6   helping with measuring changes in behaviour and feelings.

Hass–Cohen (2006) describes art therapy as a relational therapy and says that it "produces sensory integrated experiences which facilitate change and safely counterbalance traumatic environmental experiences; with simple and novel art activities which can be experienced by the amygdala as interpersonally safe, and which help provide distraction and relief from stress" (p. 10).

Brain and nervous system development

> Neuroscience involves the study of the nervous system at a molecular, cellular, and systems level.
>
> (O'Kelly, 2016, p. 1)

Developments in neuroscience have opened greater possibilities of understanding how the brain works, how it is affected by trauma of various kinds, and how it can continue to change and grow throughout the life span. They have added scientific evidence to the perspective of change as a fundamental part of therapy and added to philosophy about meaning and change throughout the life span. The use of neuroimaging has established key functions and activities of the brain. A major concept is that of brain plasticity, indicating that brain function can continue to change throughout the life span and that as new neurons develop, connections can be strengthened and further developed to perform specific functions or replace neurons which are no longer optimally functional.

Recent developments in brain imaging techniques and recognition of the role of hormones, such as cortisol in stress, have increased knowledge about the working of the brain and nervous system, including the autonomic and peripheral nervous systems. Schematic models of brain development and function have direct significance for the arts therapies, which are inherently creative, embodied, and multifaceted approaches to therapy. The imaging material from neuroscience reinforces philosophical and theoretical models, including Siegel (2012) linking mind and body with mindfulness techniques; Porges (2003), with polyvagal theory; and Schore (2005, 2009, 2014, 2019). Schore's extensive work on attachment and affect regulation refers to Bowlby's work on how early social environment interacts with the developing child to shape developmental processes. Schore (2000) says that "Bowlby presented his model in such a way that both a heuristic theoretical perspective and a testable experimental methodology could be created to observe, measure, and evaluate certain specific mechanisms by which the early social environment interacts with the maturing organism in order to shape developmental processes" (p. 24). Schore's continuing work focuses on the effects of the environment on the development of emotions and development of the right brain, and on the functions of affect regulation.

Information about how the brain develops can be utilised to design therapy to match appropriate stages and to match current developmental level, or to utilise findings about brain plasticity, mirror neurons, implicit and explicit memory, and regulatory functions for emotion and action in order to target therapy to repair and growth. Most clients presenting to therapy have experienced some environmental, social, or emotional harm to their healthy emotional development. The effects of these are planted in the brain.

Brain development

A very schematic representation of brain development is given by Hass-Cohen and Findlay (2015), with the brain developing to greater complexity from the reptilian lower brain, the limbic-central brain, and the neocortex (p. 24). These three areas represent species or epigenetic development, as well as individual human development. They also represent many human reactions to the world of senses, emotions, thoughts, and events so that a response to any sensory stimulus, through the skin, smell, and hearing, for example, may first be recognised by the lower brain and then gain further recognition and identification as information is transmitted to the other main brain regions.

Hass-Cohen and Findlay (2015) further differentiate the function of the three regions with the lower or reptilian brain being associated with motor function and sensory inputs. This region includes the spinal cord, brainstem, cerebellum, medulla, midbrain, pons, and reticular activating system.

The limbic system or central brain generates emotion and contains the amygdala, basal ganglia, hippocampus, hypothalamus, thalamus, and nucleus accumbens.

The higher brain is concerned with affect regulation and meaning-making, higher-order thinking, reason, and speech processes, and the processing of emotions and sensory information (Hass-Cohen & Findlay, 2015, p. 34).

Prendiville (2017) summarises brain functions as follows:

- The 'reptilian brain' (brainstem and cerebellum) coordinates basic regulatory functions, reflexes, level of arousal, cardiovascular functions (brainstem), and motor, emotional and cognitive functions (cerebellum).
- The 'mammalian brain' (limbic system or emotional brain) is the source of urges, needs, and feelings.
- The 'rational brain' (neocortex) is the higher part of the brain where thinking, planning and problem solving occur. It also provides for self-awareness, imagination and creativity, and empathy (p. 14).

Important roles are played by the autonomic nervous system (ANS), with sympathetic and parasympathetic and enteric subsystems. For example, the polyvagal theory of Porges (2003) is particularly influential, providing explanatory power to support several practices. The ANS has multiple interconnections with the limbic system and works to achieve homeostasis. Sensory and somatic systems, along with hormonal systems, contribute to the working of the whole brain and nervous system with constant communication between all parts of the system.

The arts therapies informed by neurodevelopment and neuroscience

Hass-Cohen and Findlay (2015) link developmental levels with targeted art therapy after assessing where emotional and neurological development might appear to have been arrested or disrupted. Play therapists also adjust play or play therapy to match developmental play as it presents rather than as age-related.

Given that the brain develops sequentially, from the lower brain towards the cortex, Prendiville and Howard (2017, p. 2) write of top-down or bottom-up approaches to therapy with playful engagement inviting relationship at a safe level (p. 7) and, citing a caution from Perry and Pate (1994), that "talking cannot translate into changes in the midbrain or the brainstem, the very areas that mediate a range of physiological, hyperactivity, behavioural impulsivity, hypervigilance, anxiety, emotional lability and sleep problems" (pp. 7, 19). Beaudoin (2017) similarly states, "In other words, controlling intense emotions with reason alone has limited effectiveness. It is more helpful to assist clients in replacing an intense physiological reaction with another, rather than cognitively attempting to stop it" (p. 82).

Working with implicit/explicit memory where trauma has occurred preverbally, the trauma cannot be named or recognised. This trauma can be transformed through imaginative play into words which can explain and alter recognition and understanding of current, otherwise mystifying feelings and behaviour, which have their origin in early trauma. Feelings and behaviours can be given names, in the present, which can give an individual some understanding of, and power over, feelings which have overwhelmed them.

Gerhardt (2004) describes the brain as being shaped by the environment, including experiences which may be emotional and nutritional or chemical. She connects common psychological difficulties in later life with the experience of non-optimal environments during the earliest development of the brain. Those commonly seen by therapists relate to self-perception, emotional resources and responsibility, ability to feel empathy for others, and depression and anxiety.

Perry outlines his essential 6 Rs for therapy with children with neurodevelopmental problems in an interview with McKinnon (2012). The 6Rs are relational, relevant, repetitive, rewarding, rhythmic, and respectful. The embodiment–projection–role paradigm of Jennings (2011) provides an earlier model for working with play and dramatherapy and with play and metaphor, along with Cattanach's model of dramatic play (1994, p. 134). Each of these facilitates communication between hemispheres.

Research relating to neuroscience and the arts therapies

Neuroscience is the scientific study of the form and functions of the brain and nervous system. Writers working with the arts therapies find strong support in neuroscience. They often work with models of brain development to see where trauma and lack of appropriate stimulation may have resulted in deficits in brain and neural development.

Hass-Cohen and Findlay (2015) align various neurological reactions with specific art therapy practices. With a particular interest in relational neurobiology, they are working towards defining specific art practices targeting neuropsychological capacities relating to making meaning, embodiment, attachment, and neuroplasticity, utilising relational co-regulation and co-creation. Their models include autobiographical memory, expressive communicating, interpersonal touch and the use of space, fear and stress, secure remembrance, transformative integrating: creating, mentalising and connecting, mindful awareness, empathy, and compassion. They have created treatment models based on art and neuroscience and developed training models for therapists to learn to work with these. They focus especially on the idea of brain plasticity to develop and strengthen neural networks, especially in working with interpersonal relationships and with strengthening neural links, following brain development models. Relational neuroscience offers a scientific basis for working with mirror neurons or following a model of working from lower brain arts activities to the higher cortex level to provide integration opportunities which have been disrupted or not developed or are not available in this situation.

In dance/movement therapy and dramatherapy, it is common to start a session with a warm-up. In both cases, this is generally physical and designed to foster an attunement of the individual with themselves and with the space they are in. In groups, a progression is often a mirroring activity during which gross and then finer movements are mirrored back to a partner. This can progress to a more intimate mirroring of a partner's facial expressions. Berrol (2006) in DMT links neural structures connected to mirror neurons to the development of empathy, attachment, attunement, social cognition, and morality. She further notes that mirror neurons can be activated in observing emotion or activity in another person as well as in personal experience. The neuroscience of mirror neurons gives scientific backing to established therapy practice, with a clear rationale of why that is effective, particularly in bringing a group together or in establishing an individual therapeutic relationship.

Homman (2010) looked at embodied concepts of neurobiology in DMT and the impact of DMT in affective neuroscience, using three vignettes to illustrate these. Referring also to body/mind connections, she references Porges (2009) for polyvagal regulation and Damasio (1999) on the concept of somatic markers, along with the work of several writers on the relevance of mirror neurons.

In dramatherapy, Dunne (2017) finds three central Narradrama processes – dramatic embodiment, dramatic projection, and distancing – provide the link between dramatherapy and neural networks, with repetition, using preferred roles, positive emotional arousal, finding unique outcomes through externalisation work, novelty, and careful focus of attention can change the structure of the brain (p. 63). Repetition and new experience work with the plasticity of the brain, while dramatic embodiment, dramatic projection, and distancing can enlarge the impact of these experiences. Frydman (2016) considers components of role theory to relate to executive function in the brain. The role system stimulates working memory. Attention, cognitive control, role definition, and theory of mind involve components of executive functioning.

Falletti (2017) considering theatre and neuroscience describes the theatre as a shared space of action, with personal space, interpersonal space, peripersonal space (p. 8) "in theatre . . . audience and actor are creating a dynamic shared space of action" also "has emotional brain resonance through mirror neurons" which "fire in resonance with the actions of others" (p. 12).

Umiltà (2017) says that in the theatre, "observing a motor act causes an automatic activation in the observer of the same neural mechanism triggered by the execution of a similar motor act" (p. 16). Theatre provides "social cognition: by sharing the same mind-body system of the individuals we face, we gain automatic access to their internal world" (p. 22).

She claims that there are

> three particularly important elements for theatrology: the direct link between mechanisms of perception and the motor system (between perception and action), the concept of consciousness as a circular process between the human body and the environment, and the obsolescence of the logical dichotomy between interior and exterior. . . .

and

> each time we perceive an action, it resonates in our body-mind system which 'translates' the action according to our motor and biographical baggage, our learning systems, and our cultural conditioning.
>
> (p. 51)

For music therapy, Sena Moore (2013) reviewed literature on the neural effects of music on emotion regulation, with emotional regulation (ER) defined as an "internal process which maintains a comfortable state of arousal by modulating states of arousal" (p. 198). ER is characterised by increased activation in the cognitive control and monitoring areas – the anterior cingulate cortex, orbitofrontal cortex, and lateral prefrontal cortex – which leads to decreased activation of the amygdala. Overall "results indicated that there are certain music characteristics and music experiences that produce such activation patterns" (Sena Moore, 2013, p. 198). Focus and attention were found to be important for example, "instruct the client to attend to a specific characteristic of the music (e.g., the melodic line, a musical cue, etc.), thus removing their focus from the emotional event" (Sena Moore, 2013, p. 235).

O'Kelly (2016) reviewed the effects of music therapy linked with neuroscience with diverse clinical populations. He cites research where music therapy was used in motor rehabilitation, affective disorders, stroke, cancer and palliative care, disorders of consciousness, and autism spectrum disorders. This is a rich field where neuroscientific technology, such as fMRI (functional magnetic resonance imaging), PET (positron emission tomography), EEG (electroencephalogram), and DTI (diffusion tensor imaging) have been used. He reports on studies on singing using biomarkers relating to stress, immunity, or social affiliation, which indicated reduction in stress and arousal; and chemical and hormonal tests which have been used to locate and confirm the effects of music therapy. "As a consequence of these collaborations, neuroscientific understanding is emerging of how music therapy may support improvements in cognition, movement and emotional regulation, as well as helping us to explore the neurological aspects of therapeutic relationships" (O'Kelly, 2016, p. 1). He cautions against using these findings as "reductive explanations of clinical work", saying that "neuroscience methods should be used concurrently with clinical markers of progress, and research methods which serve the qualitative, experiential, and relational aspects of music therapy" (O'Kelly, 2016, p. 11).

Ward (1999) considers process in art therapy in the relationship of the client to the material. She says, "The way that someone relates to a medium through their body language can become the mirror for their being. How the body is used is a powerful message to the therapist of an individual's state of mind" and "the actual physical struggle and contact between the medium and the body is so important because it is through the struggle that creative solutions are often found" (Ward, 1999, p. 111).

Art therapists and creative arts therapies/expressive arts therapies have explored neuroscience links over many years. Lusebrink (2004) developed the expressive therapies continuum (ETC) as a model for a series of art therapy sessions. Activities involve different motor, somatosensory, visual, emotional, and cognitive aspects of information processing with corresponding neurophysiological processes and brain structures. She arranged activities and materials as perceived through tactile-haptic and visual, sensory, and perceptual channels. She described interactions with media and expressions created in art therapy, on three different levels of complexity – kinaesthetic/sensory, perceptual/affective, and cognitive/symbolic. A fourth level, the creative level, she conceptualised as crossing the other levels (Lusebrink, 2004, p. 129). Hinz (2015) demonstrates the use of the ETC, illustrated with case study material. She provides a clear explanation of ETC and the "way in which clients interact with various media in art therapy is hypothesised to parallel the ways they process information in other areas of their lives" (Hinz, 2015, p. 43). This gives an indication of starting points for therapy.

Kaimal et al. (2016) found changes in cortisol levels following artmaking. In a quasi-experimental study on the impact of artmaking on cortisol levels of 39 healthy adults, they found that the mean cortisol levels were lower for 75% of the sample after artmaking. "There were weak to moderate correlations between the lowering of cortisol and the narrative response themes of learning about self and the evolving process of art making" (Kaimal et al., 2016, p. 13).

> "The arts are neuropsychology in action" (Zaidel, 2005, cited in King et al., 2019, p. 149).
>
> Advances in the field of neuroscience can be used to support scientific research and best practices in the profession of art therapy. Integrating neuroscience research into our practice . . . can complement arts-based research that calls on intuition and phenomenological evidence that contributes to the holism of the profession.
>
> King et al. (2019, p. 154)

> Kaimal et al. (2016) in a quasi-experimental study found "that art making resulted in statistically significant lowering of cortisol levels."
>
> (p. 74)

King et al. (2019) say that artmaking integrates visual, emotional, and behavioural outputs. Art therapy integrates cognitive, emotional, and relational elements to induce or support change (King et al., 2019, p. 150) and while "Many art therapists might be content employing the broad concept that art can provide a key to unlocking memories, feelings, and therapeutic insights . . . a more accurate understanding of brain structures involved with cognitive and emotional processing can support intentional clinical choice" (King et al., 2019, p. 15). Konopka (2014) adds that "we already know that art therapy leads to reframing experiences, reorganizing thoughts and gaining personal insights, while adding neuroscience has the potential to validate effects on brain function and theoretically to target therapy" (p. 73).

For many years, Malchiodi (2012, 2014, 2020a, 2020b, 2020c) has tracked research and writing on the approaches of art and expressive therapies for working with traumatised adults and children, particularly the "[i]mportance of early attachment on neurological functions throughout life; and the impact of trauma on memory" (p. 17). She says, "Art making is an experience that can simultaneously engage many parts of the brain including the cortical (symbolizing, decision making, and planning), the limbic (affect and emotion), and the midbrain/brainstem (sensory and kinaesthetic) systems" (p. 19) and "posttraumatic stress disorder (PTSD) is defined through both psychological and physiological symptoms" (p. 21).

"Art is a natural sensory mode of expression because it involves touch, smell, and other senses within the experience." Art therapy has "attachment and relational aspects. All Creative Arts Therapies offer relational mirroring, role play, enactment, sharing, showing, and witnessing" Malchiodi (2005) and "In Art therapy . . . interaction (is) through experiential, tactile, and visual exchanges, not just verbal communication, between the client and the therapist."

Malchiodi (2020b) outlines Porges' polyvagal theory (2011), in which the ventral vagal network that runs from the diaphragm to the brain stem has a key importance because it can be influenced by breathing patterns and social cues such as smiling and making eye contact to generate a sense of calm and safety from over-arousal. Malchiodi (2020b) writes of the role of rhythmic synchronisation, humming, and vocal toning as examples to connect with this system to aid emotional regulation (pp. 2–3).

A major disruptor of healthy neurological development is exposure to violence, particularly in childhood. Perry (1997) says an effect of this disruption at a crucial stage of development can predispose to violence by decreasing the strength of the subcortical and cortical impulse-modulating capacity and by decreasing the value of other humans due to an incapacity to empathise or sympathise with them (p. 131). This underlines the value of intervention at a neurological level. Describing a neurosequential model of therapeutics, Perry and Hambrick (2008) say,

> The more the therapeutic process can replicate the normal sequential process of development, the more effective the interventions are. Simply stated, the idea is to start with the lowest (in the brain) undeveloped/abnormally functioning set of problems and move sequentially up the brain as improvements are seen.
>
> (p. 42)

Conclusion

Kapitan (2014) describes the introduction of neurobiology to art therapy, "as evidence-based, complex, and influential" (p. 1).

Particular features of neuroscience which are relevant to therapists include the sequential development of the brain, the specialisation of areas of the brain, brain plasticity, and other features like mirror neurons which have been identified as active in interpersonal relationships.

Beaudoin (2017) says, "Neuron cells have the neuroplastic ability to learn and are therefore particularly vulnerable to being shaped by experience" (p. 75).

Learning from neuroscience has the capacity to further inform and shape our practice in the arts therapies. There is much more that arts therapists can learn and adapt from neuroscience. O'Kelly (2016) has said that findings from neuroscience add to the practice of the arts therapies by aligning with current practices. They do not constitute an imposition of science onto practice of the arts therapies. Rather, they add rationale for their use and clarification of their efficacy. They are not reductionist; neither do they present a single more important view to the theoretical and philosophical bases of the arts therapies. They add explanatory power to the way the arts therapies are practised, and to the effects seen in practice, and allow the possibility of adding another dimension to the planning of work with clients (O'Kelly, 2016, p. 1).

Some other writers, while embracing what neuroscience has to offer to therapists, also sound a note of caution about what is relevant and how it is used. Strong (2017) says, "Helping clients recognize that particular interactions have a greater chance of recurring because they also concurrently activate brain processes is different from suggesting that their brains are responsible for empathy or sharing" (p. 120). He cautions against making causal inferences but encourages the use of knowledge of neuroscience alongside established ways of working (Strong, 2017, p. 124).

Beaudoin and Duvall (2017) add that "lived experiences were finally recognized as being both shaped by, *and shaping of*, the brain" (p. 6) and, citing Siegel (2007), "[s]imply put, the mind influences the brain, which affects relationships, which in turn affect the mind" (p. 7).

> Neuroscience continues to provide an ever-widening understanding of how the brain and body react to stress, trauma, illness, and other events. It also is central to understanding how images influence emotions, thoughts, and well-being and how the visual, sensory, and expressive language of art are best integrated into treatment.
>
> (Malchiodi, 2012, p. 24)

Findings from neuroscience both confirm the existing principles and ways of working with the arts therapies and suggest new ways of working. Relational neuroscience underlines the importance all therapists place on building a safe and trusting relationship with clients, as the firm basis of any future work. Neuroscience confirms the importance of the additional elements the arts bring to therapeutic relationships and particularly the nature of embodiment inherent in all the arts therapies with its specific relationship to neuroscience and the neurological systems of the brain and body. Mind and body are intrinsically linked, and the reactions and emotions of the body can now be understood in a different and expanded way through the practical implications of neuroscience.

Acknowledgements

With many thanks to Payal working in Delhi, dealing with all our queries in a timely way, while living in a sea of COVID-19, which had seemed to be disappearing and then returned with a vengeance.

Many warm thanks to all the writers who presented their worlds and their views and their wonderful work so this book could be written. You have all been incredibly patient in writing, rewriting, discussing, looking with new eyes, and producing subtly different approaches, practices, and views of the arts therapies arising from your own training, culture, and life and work environments. Your willingness to learn from neuroscience has been inspiring.

Thanks to Mariana and Bruce Torkington for their work on all the images and to Mariana for editorial support throughout the development of the book.

References

Beaudoin, M. (2017). Helping clients thrive with positive emotions: Expanding people's repertoire of problem counter-states. In M. Beaudoin & J. Duvall (Eds.), *Collaborative therapy and neurobiology: Evolving practices in action* (pp. 28–39). Routledge.

Beaudoin, M. N., & Duvall, J. (Eds.). (2017). *Collaborative therapy and neurobiology: Evolving practices in action*. Routledge.

Berrol, C. F. (2006). Neuroscience meets dance/movement therapy: Mirror neurons, the therapeutic process and empathy. *The Arts in Psychotherapy, 33*(4), 302–315. https://doi.org/10.1016/j.aip.2006.04.001

Cattanach, A. (1994). Dramatic play with children: The interface of dramatherapy and play-therapy. Ch. 8. In S. Jennings, A. Cattanach, S. Mitchell, A. Chesner, & B. Meldrum (Eds.), *The handbook of dramatherapy*. Routledge.

Csikszentmihalyi, M. (1996). *Creativity flow and the psychology of discovery and invention*. Harper Perennial.

Damasio, A. (1999). *The feeling of what happens: Body and emotion in the making of consciousness*. Harcourt College Publishers.

Dunne, P. (2017). Insights on positive change an exploration of the link between drama-therapy and neural networks. Chp. 5. In M. Beaudoin & J. Duvall (Eds.), *Collaborative therapy and neurobiology: Evolving practices in action*. Routledge.

Falletti, C. (2017). The shared space of action. Introduction. In C. Falletti, G. Sofia, & V. Jacona (Eds.), *Theatre and cognitive neuroscience*. Bloomsbury.

Frydman, J. S. (2016). Role theory and executive functioning: Constructing cooperative paradigms of drama therapy and cognitive neuropsychology. *The Arts in Psychotherapy, 47*, 41–47.

Gerhardt, S. (2004). *Why love matters: How affection shapes a baby's brain*. Routledge.

Hass-Cohen, N. (2006). Art therapy and clinical neuroscience in action. *GAINS Community Newsletter*, 10–12.

Hass-Cohen, N., & Findlay, J. C. (2015). *Art therapy & the neuroscience of relationships, creativity, & resiliency*. W. W. Norton.

Hinz, L. D. (2015). Expressive therapies continuum: Use and value demonstrated with case study. *Canadian Art Therapy Association Journal, 28*(1–2), 43–50.

Homman, K. B. (2010). Embodied concepts of neurobiology in dance/movement therapy practice. *American Journal of Dance Therapy, 32*(2), 80–99.

Jennings, S. (2011). *Healthy attachments and neuro-dramatic play*. Jessica Kingsley.

Kaimal, K., Ray, K., & Muniz, J. (2016). Reduction of cortisol levels and participants' responses following art making. *Art Therapy, 33*(2), 74–80. doi:1080/07421656.2016.1166832

Kapitan, L. (2014). Introduction to the neurobiology of art therapy: Evidence based, complex, and influential. *Art Therapy: Journal of the American Art Therapy Association, 3*(2), 50–51.

King, J. L., Kaimal, G., Konopka, L., Belkofer, C., & Strang, C. (2019). Practical applications of neuroscience-informed art therapy. *Art Therapy: Journal of the American Art Therapy Association, 36*(3), 149–156.

Konopka, L. M. (2014). Where art meets neuroscience: A new horizon of art therapy. *Croatian Medical Journal, 55*(1), 73–74. doi.10.3325/cmi.2014.55.73

Kottman, T., Dickinson, R., & Meany-Walen, K. (2017). The role of non-directive and directive/focused approaches to play and expressive arts therapy for children, adolescents and adults. In E. Prendiville & J. Howard (Eds.), *Creative psychotherapy: Applying the principles of neurobiology and expressive arts–based practice* (p. 51). Routledge.

Lusebrink, V. B. (2004). Art therapy and the brain: An attempt to understand the underlying processes of art expression in therapy. *Art Therapy: Journal of the American Art Therapy Association, 21*(3), 125–135.

Malchiodi, C. A. (2005). Expressive therapies, history, theory and practice. Chp. 2. In C. Malchiodi (Ed.), *Expressive therapies*. Guilford Publications.

Malchiodi, C. A. (2012). Art therapy and the brain. Chp. 2. In C. Malchiodi (Ed.), *Handbook of art therapy* (2nd ed.). Guilford Press.

Malchiodi, C. A. (2014). Creative arts therapy approaches to attachment issues. In C. Malchiodi & D. Crenshaw (Eds.), *Creative arts and play therapy for attachment problems* (pp. 3–18). Guilford Press.

Malchiodi, C. A. (2020a). Trauma, self-regulation, and expressive arts therapy. *Psychology Today*. www.psychologytoday.com/us/blog/arts-and-health/202001/trauma

Malchiodi, C. A. (2020b). Tapping the healing rhythms of the vagal nerve. *Psychology Today*. www.psychologytoday.com/us/blog/arts-and-health/202004/tapping

Malchiodi, C. A. (2020c). *Trauma and expressive arts therapy: Brain, body, and imagination in the healing process*. Guilford Press.

McGrath, E. (2017). The role of music and rhythm in the development, integration and repair of the self. Chp. 5. In E. Prendiville & J. Howard (Eds.), *Creative psychotherapy: Applying the principles of neurobiology to play and expressive arts-based practice*. Routledge.

McKinnon, L. (2012). The neurosequential model of therapeutics: An interview with Bruce Perry. *Australian and New Zealand Journal of Family Therapy, 33*(3), 210–218.

O'Kelly, J. (2016). Music therapy and neuroscience: Opportunities and challenges. *Voices A World Forum for Music Therapy*. https://doi.org/10.15845/voices.v16i2.872.172

Perry, B. D. (1997). Incubated in terror: Neurodevelopmental factors in the "cycle of violence". In J. D. Osofsky (Ed.), *Children in a violent society* (pp. 124–148). Guilford Publications.

Perry, B. D., & Hambrick, E. P. (2008). The neurosequential model of therapeutics. *Reclaiming Children and Youth, 17*(3), 38–43.

Perry, B. D., & Pate, J. (1994). Neurodevelopment and the psychobiological roots of post-traumatic stress disorder. In L. Koziol & C. Stout (Eds.), *The neuropsychology of mental disorders: A practical guide* (pp. 129–146). Charles C. Thomas.

Pitruzzella, S. (2009). Creativity and arts therapy: A dramatherapist's perspective. In S. Scobie, M. Ross, & C. Lapoujade (Eds.), *Arts in arts therapies: A European perspective*. ECArTE.

Porges, S. W. (2003). The polyvagal theory: Phylogenetic contributions to social behaviour. *Physiology and behaviour, 79*, 503–513.

Porges, S. W. (2009). Reciprocal influences between body and brain in the perception and expression of affect: A polyvagal perspective. In D. Fosha, D. J. Siegel, & M. F. Solomon (Eds.), *The healing power of emotion: Affective neuroscience, development, clinical practice*. W. W. Norton.

Porges, S. W. (2011). *The polyvagal theory: Neurophysiological foundations of emotions, attachment, communication, and self-regulation* (pp. 27-54). W.W. Norton Publications.

Prendiville, E. (2017). Neurobiology for psychotherapists. Chp. 1. In E. Prendiville & J. Howard, (Eds.), *Creative psychotherapy: Applying the principles of neurobiology and expressive arts-based practice*. Routledge.

Prendiville, E., & Howard, J. (2017). *Creative psychotherapy: Applying the principles of neurobiology and expressive arts-based practice*. Routledge.

Schore, A. N. (2000). Attachment and the regulation of the right brain. *Attachment & Human Development, 2*(1), 23–47.

Schore, A. N. (2005). Back to basics: Attachment, affect regulation, and the developing right brain: Linking developmental neuroscience to paediatrics. *Paediatrics in Review, 26*(6), 204–217. https://doi.org/10.1542/pir.26-6-204

Schore, A. N. (2014). Early interpersonal neurobiological assessment of attachment and autistic spectrum disorders. *Frontiers in Psychology, 5,* 1–13. doi:103389/fpsyg. 2014.01049

Schore, A. N. (2009). Relational trauma and the developing right brain: An interface of psychoanalytic self-psychology and neuroscience. *Annals of the New York Academy of Science, 1159,* 189–203. doi:10.1111/j.1749-6632i.2009.04474.xschore

Schore, A. N. (2019). *Right brain psychotherapy*. Norton Professional Books.

Sena Moore, K. (2013). A systematic review on the neural effects of music on emotion regulation: Implications for music therapy practice. *Journal of Music Therapy, 50*(3), 198–242.

Siegel, D. J. (2007). *The mindful brain*. W.W. Norton and Company.

Siegel, D. J. (2012). Mind, brain and relationships: The interpersonal neurobiology perspective. In *The developing mind: How relationships and the brain interact to shape who we are* (2nd ed.). Guilford Press.

Strong, T. (2017). Neuroscience discourse and the collaborative therapies? Chp. 9. In M. Beaudoin & J. Duvall (Eds.), *Collaborative therapy and neurobiology Evolving practices in action.* Routledge.

Umiltà, M. A. (2017). The 'mirror mechanism' and motor behaviour. Chp. 1. In C. Falletti, G. Sofia, & V. Jacona (Eds.), *Theatre and cognitive neuroscience*. Bloomsbury.

Ward, C. (1999). Shaping connections hands-on art therapy. In A. Cattanach (Ed.), *Process in the arts therapies* (pp.103-131). Jessica Kingsley.

Part II

Arts therapies in practice

2 Exploring implicit memory through metaphor

Jonah and the missing heart: a story of attachment and dramatherapy

Sarah Mann Shaw

Introduction

Jonah was a four-and-a-half-year-old boy of mixed heritage with a black British Caribbean mother and white British father. The following case study examines the roles of metaphor and neuroscience, attachment, and trauma within dramatherapy.

People from a former British colony in the Caribbean, immigrated to the United Kingdom mainly in the 1950s to fill labour gaps; many were descendants of slaves. Later generations became crucial workers in health and care, as well as in building and infrastructure projects. They are still often in low paid work in inner-city areas, bearing the stresses of poverty and discrimination. There is considerable intermarriage. As a white therapist, I was culturally sensitive and aware that I was working with a mixed-race family.

Background

The explicit story

Through dramatherapy assessment processes (Mann Shaw, 2016), the explicit story is gathered from the client, significant others, written records, reports, and any support systems. The explicit story is that which is known and held in conscious memory and is coherent and sequential in nature. It is recalled and verbalised intentionally "through the engagement of the cortical systems of the brain" (Carey, 2017, p. 44). Jonah's age and early trauma experiences meant he was unlikely to have access to a clear verbal narrative of his experience. Van der Kolk (1998, cited in Carey, 2017) writes that as fear increases, access to the language centre of the brain goes off-line, as we react to sensory cues in the environment and within our body. The adults around Jonah provided the explicit story, the timeline of his early experiences.

Jonah's birth mother had experienced perinatal depression during her pregnancy with his older brother, and had attempted suicide. Jonah's father had a history of threatening behaviour, violence, cannabis use, and a diagnosis of anti-social personality disorder. The family had been referred to a child protection service.

DOI: 10.4324/9781003082897-6

Over the six months following Jonah's birth, further referrals to child protection services related to Jonah's failure to gain weight, domestic violence and verbal abuse, and the mother's difficulty in complying with antidepressant medication. Jonah was moved into foster care at the age of 13 months after further reports of neglect and admission to hospital after his father threw boiling water at his mother while she was holding him. When Jonah came to dramatherapy, he had been in foster care for three years and was now living with his adoptive parents, whose cultural heritage reflected that of his birth parents.

The implicit story

The implicit story of Jonah's early experience was in his visual, olfactory, auditory, kinaesthetic, non-verbal experience. This is connected to the amygdala, is emotionally driven, is hypersensitive to external stimuli, and is connected to trauma. It relates to the limbic system and can affect an individual's capacity to regulate emotion and feel safe in relationships (Dana, 2018). Dana (2018) explains that "trauma compromises our ability to engage with others, by replacing patterns of connection with patterns of protection" (p. xviii). My work with Jonah focused on how to safely externalise his trauma story, moving from a range of sensory experiences into a conscious realm of reference without re-traumatising him. This meant keeping Jonah safe and curious about his own story while giving him a language to process and experience his life differently.

When early experience has been characterised by neglect and violence, the development of the right hemisphere is compromised, causing difficulties with responding to social environments appropriately and regulating emotions. This can create an intolerable sense of feeling overwhelmed or unconsciously dissociating from emotions to prevent them from reaching awareness. Repair is created by restructuring the emotional brain through building new neural networks. Achieving this requires an emotionally attuned and playful therapeutic process. Wilkinson (2010) writes that the therapist must pay careful attention to the flow of attachment and separation and be open to the client's nonverbal cues and emotional states. A secure attachment to the therapist "activates key drivers of neuroplasticity, such as decreases in cortisol, which inhibits hippocampal functioning, protein synthesis, and new learning" (Cozolino, 2017, p. 58). This level of attunement necessitates working in a right-brained mode and requires a reflective approach in the therapist, a wondering about the play and the character's dilemma. The more I modelled reflective curiosity about Jonah's play, the more he was enabled to reflect and explore meaning in his character's experiences.

Jonah's mirror neurons could be sensitive to my intentions and feelings in our relationship. As I modelled empathy, enquiry, and responsiveness to his story, he felt safer and more emotionally open. Mirror neurons as a mechanism regulate interpersonal relations via a process of simulation, at a pre-reflective, pre-cognitive level. This generates a shared space of action, the same state of motor, corporeal and emotive change in actor and spectator. This double-activation pattern is an embodied simulation which, in turn, produces an interpersonal attuned intention that establishes resonance. The response is immediate rather than processed or presumed by areas of higher cortical processes. Comprehension is immediate. I understand because I am simply redoing the same action I see before me. "A brain which acts is also and above all a brain which understands" (Rizzolatti & Sinigaglia, 2008, p. 9).

Attachment

Children like Jonah, who have experienced insecure attachments, may develop a capacity for self-sufficiency without a predictable and consistent adult to help them understand and manage troublesome feelings.

Attachment theories (Bowlby, 1982; Fahlberg, 1991; Howe, 2005) and the impact of trauma (Crenshaw, 2014; Perry, 2009; Schore, 2013; Siegel, 2001; Van der Kolk, 2005, 2014), which hinder a child's capacity for relational development are important foundations for working with children with a history of neglect. These early relationships have a profound impact on the structure of our emotional brain, our relationship with our self and with others, and on our sense of psychological well-being.

Early experiences of neglect and violence may compromise the development of the right hemisphere, producing difficulty responding to social environments appropriately and in regulating our emotions. This can create feelings of being overwhelmed, which can become intolerable. Dissociation is a defence mechanism that has a protective function, preventing emotions from reaching awareness.

Achieving changes in neural networks requires an emotionally attuned and playful therapeutic process. Winnicott (2005) referenced the importance of the mother–child, patient–therapist bond and the need for the mother/therapist to create a 'holding environment' that enables play which allows further opportunity for healthy neurodevelopment. Engaging in therapeutic play may reveal aspects of the child's inner world: their thoughts, their feelings, and their preoccupations which may affect their attachment behaviours. Their stories also give clues to the imaginative material which can help in their healing. A child's capacity to emotionally regulate comes from their interpersonal experiences. Through secure attachment, with a significant adult, children learn to regulate their emotions and to name and manage their feelings. When a child's significant other has had limited capacity to name the child's affect, the child will have less capacity for self-regulation. Where there have also been traumatic experiences, the child will have a greater propensity for psychological defences such as dissociation (Irwin, 2005).

Basis of practice

Irwin (2005) writes that most dramatherapists work towards a facilitation of imaginative play, a strengthening of self-regulation and self-control, and supporting clients to put feelings into words. This work is facilitated through a metaphorical narrative that dramatherapist and client engage in, creating, playing, and exploring together. We are working with a containing metaphor for our clients' stories. "Abstract notions are tied to our bodies through metaphor, thus connecting our minds to the world through the experience of our bodies" (Cozolino, 2006, p. 73). Johnson (2000) writes that playing with the metaphor and developing it into a coherent narrative supports the child to express that which is inexpressible and to begin to find meaning and language to make sense of experience. Dramatherapists will make enquiries about the child's play as it unfolds, looking out for pertinent themes, difficulties, and capacities for problem-solving, paying careful attention to material presented through embodiment (implicit) and that which is presented through verbal narration (explicit), and being open to the way the child chooses to tell their story. If a child cannot access a helping character in their metaphorical narrative this may imply a difficulty in trusting another as a reliable source of help. This suggests another area to develop in the play.

Initial meetings and assessment

Jonah's adoptive parents explained that they felt something was '*wrong with Jonah*'. They described him as '*noisy, resistant to instructions and very active*' with some unusual behaviours that might indicate underlying developmental or learning issues. His teacher and the special educational needs coordinator described him as '*noisy and aggressive*' and were concerned about Jonah's capacity to '*focus and learn*'. The adoptive parents felt they had not initially been given an accurate description of Jonah's difficulties and felt angry and frustrated about being '*hoodwinked*'.

We agreed that Jonah's adoptive mother would attend the sessions in the role of observer unless Jonah made a specific request for her help. She agreed to follow his play, resisting interpretations or direct questions. I explained that children's metaphoric play may contain multiple meanings and that to attach a single meaning might inhibit the expansive nature of play. Jonah, himself, might attach specific meanings which we would note (Fonagy, 2004). We might imagine what the meaning felt like for him. She agreed and expressed a real interest in witnessing Jonah's play.

I offered a six-week assessment block (Mann Shaw, 2016) which follows a developmental model of embodiment, projection, and role (Jennings, 2011). This model focuses on engagement with dramatic play to help understand the child's inner world, worries, preoccupations, and capacity to use the resources available, including the role of helper/guide or wise person and the relationship with the dramatherapist. The therapist follows the child's lead, with curious enquiry and playing roles assigned by the child. The role of witness is also crucial (Jones, 2007) to act as an audience to the drama, the client, and/or to oneself as therapist or player.

Arriving for his first session, Jonah walked ahead of his mother (adoptive) and confidently entered the therapy room, smiling at me and asking about the toys. I had prepared PSYCHLOPS for Kids (Haythorne et al., 2012), as an age-appropriate assessment measure. Jonah could not engage with this but later named his presenting problem as '*mummy being cross*'.

The main assessment was therefore based on the Embodiment, Projection and Role paradigm (Jennings, 2011) through 'tracking', referring to the dramatherapist's ability to create resonance (Schore, 2013) in the therapeutic relationship; to make appropriate enquiry about the characters, themes, and direction of the child's dramatic play; and to work to the developmental presentation of the child. At this stage in Jonah's dramatherapy, his play was largely projective and involved creating small worlds and objects to narrate a story. Symbolic play supports the use of creativity to solve problems, to self-regulate, and to experience delight and mutual exploration.

I sat on the floor next to Jonah, while his mother remained on the sofa keeping an interested eye on his play. Jonah was immediately drawn to a box of puppets and picked a black finger puppet, naming it Jonah. Gersie (1992) advocates a story structure, in which the narrative is developed along the lines of character, location, potential threat/difficulty, helper, engagement with difficulty, and resolution. Jonah created a home where little black Jonah could live with his mother. A brave knight was invited to join them; however, the knight had a volatile temper and stabbed puppet Jonah's heart. I wondered aloud how this was for puppet Jonah and suggested that it might have hurt a lot. Jonah produced a doctor's kit, saying that he was a doctor and was going to see if he could fix the puppet's heart. However, he discovered that the puppet's heart had '*gone*'. When I asked where the heart was, the doctor said, '*[I]t is at the bottom of the sea and only a diver could get it*'. I suggested that Jonah and I could make the sea together out of materials in the room, and he was keen to engage. When invited to choose an object to be the heart at the bottom of the ocean, he explained that no one could see the heart as it had '*disappeared*' and was '*too far down to see*'. I asked about a toy which might be a good deep-sea diver; Jonah took a good look and shook his head, saying, '*[N]o*'. Jonah had created an amazing metaphorical story illustrating his life situation and his continuing dilemma.

Jonah then moved to the story of the knight and the puppet Jonah, with no heart. The knight explained that when puppet Jonah was a baby, he had '*cried and cried and cried and that now*' he (the knight) was '*cross*'. Jonah introduced a black mummy puppet and gave it to me, asking me to play this role. It appeared that the problem of the Jonah puppet could not be addressed until we had considered the knight. As mummy puppet I asked the knight what would help him be less cross? The knight thought food might help and asked for porridge with raisins. This was created and offered by the mummy puppet. Jonah told me that this character was less angry but still '*cross*' and would attack puppet Jonah again. In character I explained that although she understood the knight's crossness, he would not be allowed to hurt puppet Jonah as it was her job to keep Jonah puppet safe. My thinking was that introducing the notion of a secure attachment into the play might give me some idea of Jonah's capacity to understand

and make use of this relationship in his dramatisation of this metaphor. Jonah puppet then informed the mummy puppet that sometimes his heart was in his tummy. This disclosure indicated that Jonah had some capacity to share his internal state. Jonah decided to put the knight and his porridge in a tower so that it had sustenance but could not hurt the puppet. At this point, Jonah told me that he missed Mama, his foster carer, the only explicit non-metaphorical comment he had made in the session. However, he very quickly withdrew this and said he did not miss her. Briefly he appeared to freeze, becoming disengaged with his play and with me. I reflected to Jonah that it might be hard to think about people who were missed or missing. Jonah looked at me and nodded; it felt as if he was no longer 'missing' from the session.

Reflections on the assessment sessions

Embodiment

Jonah expressed a range of feelings through the visceral images in his play/story. He displayed congruence with verbal and body expressions.

Projection

Jonah's play enabled him to project a range of feelings onto the characters, food, and habitats he created.

Role

It was noticeable that Jonah opted to represent himself within the play with a cast of fictional characters with a range of characteristics. His choices could hold clues about how he viewed his identity as a dual-heritage child.

Attachment

Jonah was able to bring a maternal figure into the play and assign it to me. I wondered if exploration and repair around this role was crucial to Jonah's therapeutic relationship and could be repaired through play and support a deepening of attachment with his adoptive mother. This aspect of his therapy was the predominant feature.

Therapy sessions

For the next session Jonah again entered the therapy space easily and began to play with his characters. I had placed the Jonah puppet and his mummy, the knight, and his tower with his porridge as Jonah had left them at the end of his first session, but he ignored them. I wondered if the play of the previous week and Jonah's disclosure at the end of the session had been too difficult for him to manage. I recalled the need for pace, allowing Jonah to retain control over his play, as he had experienced little control over decisions in his previous life.

Jonah told me he needed a castle and picked up a box of Power Rangers, arranging them around the castle. He said the Rangers had wanted to enter the castle for '*two weeks but that they were too cross*'. He added that they needed help from lots of toys to manage this. I thought about how cross Jonah might be and that he could be referring to his own need for help. He had not experienced being able to get 'inside' another, to be emotionally held and contained. Jonah said that the other toys needed a '*nice home*'. He spent most of the session arranging the inside of the castle with a seat and a bed for each ranger. He picked a black ranger as the main helper and allowed him into the castle. Once this ranger took up residence, Jonah picked up two other rangers, who knocked at the door of the castle, asking to come in.

'Are you good'? asked the black ranger.

'Yes', they replied.

'Okay', said the black ranger, letting them in.

Each ranger was tucked into a bed. The session ended, but Jonah was reluctant to leave, saying that he needed to '*play some more*'. I felt that this was an important statement, indicating a wish to make more choices and recognising that he could do this in the play space. Perhaps the creation of a safe place for the Rangers had prompted a feeling of internal safety, allowing him to feel soothed and contained as the Rangers were inside the safety of the castle. I considered the themes of Jonah's play. He again referenced crossness as a dominant affect; however, the Rangers recognised the importance of secure relationships. I wondered if Jonah was beginning to think about the importance of feeling safe and secure versus the more unpredictable and harmful relationships of the previous session.

In session four, Jonah gave the 'naughty knight' a friend so that he could learn to be less angry. It seemed that Jonah was getting a sense of being the external modulator, both in relationship with me and in the relationships between his different characters and perhaps for himself. By giving the knight a friend, Jonah had found a way of holding this aspect of his experience and offering the character help to feel more psychologically robust. Looking at my bookshelf, he asked if there were any books that could help him '*get rid of monsters*'. I responded that there might be and wondered if we could find a way of playing with monsters to make them less scary. Jonah seemed to want to know how to be less troubled by monsters and what he might experience as monstrous thoughts, feelings, and experiences. I was reminded of his history of domestic violence and assault on his body, mind, feelings, and development. I felt compassion and warmth for this little boy who had survived so much and yet remained curious.

In his next session, Jonah returned to the question of the lost heart. He picked a boxed red crystal for the heart and placed it underneath the fabric representing the sea. He manipulated a puppet to dive under the sea and collect the box. I wondered if he had remembered my suggestion of this in the first dramatherapy session. He took the box to his mum and carefully opened it to show her the lost heart. She told him how beautiful and special the heart was and how glad she was that Jonah had shown it to her. He showed courage in letting a trusted other help him manage this successfully. Jonah's play was beginning to include important themes of secure attachment; he trusted having a heart and having a reliable person to support him.

In the next session, Jonah began to explore the role of 'daddy'. He said the characters were angry because there was a big scary monster that they could not do anything about and there was a *'big scary daddy who was really loud'* who *'told all the kids to be angry'*. Jonah took a large *'scary daddy dinosaur'* who killed the Rangers and puppet Jonah, then moved towards his mother. I wondered aloud whether it intended to kill her too and how she might deal with this. She picked up on my cue, roaring at the dinosaur. Jonah manipulated it to run away and hide, grinning at his mother as he did so and soon after climbed onto her knee for a hug. Later in the session, he took the dead puppet Jonah to his mother, and she, instinctively, revived it with *'magic kisses'*. At this point, Jonah reported that he felt really tired and needed to go home. His mother reflected that fighting off scary monsters was probably a tiring business and that perhaps he needed to rest and be looked after by her.

Perhaps Jonah's internal experience of crossness masked his sadness. His previous play had been dominated by crossness. It was as if the knight, the puppet Jonah, and the Power Rangers all wanted something that they were unable to attain, experience, and internalise. The tiredness in this session was perhaps an indicator of how difficult this process was for Jonah. He was constantly in motion, legs, arms, words always prepared for action. The search for the other was constantly thwarted until his mum stepped in and demonstrated something different. In witnessing and experiencing this Jonah's posture changed, as he allowed himself to be held in his mother's arms and gaze.

Reflections

The theory of dramatic play (Emunah, 1994; Jones, 2007) suggests that in all play there is a process of dramatic projection (Jones, 2007), that in the process of play children engage in placing parts of themselves and their feelings onto objects in the play. The dramatherapist supports the child in the process and encourages the telling of a metaphorical story through symbolic objects which hold projected meaning. The dramatic play enables the child to engage with difficult themes and feelings at a safe enough distance to encourage engagement and exploration. Projection becomes expressive whereas in traditional psychotherapy, projection is sometimes seen as a defense. Dramatherapy emphasises the ways that projection can be linked to dramatic form to enable a client to create, discover, and engage with external representations of internal conflicts. Once there is a conscious and articulated story, the possibility of integrating all the previously fragmented sensory experiences exists.

Children with traumatic early-life experiences will often internalise family difficulties as being about them, feeling that if only they could be better or do things right, then the adults around them might be happier and able to meet their needs (Van der Kolk, 2005). This is not a conscious thought process. It happens at neurobiological, embodied, and relational levels. Children with secure parents experience secure attachments and grow up believing that the world is a good place and when things go wrong adults can help them. Children without these experiences have more difficulty believing that the world is a good and safe place and that difficulties, and difficult feelings, can be managed.

The need for relational containment to assimilate difficult affect became a strong theme of our continued sessions. Jonah needed to experience a safe and therapeutic relationship where trust could be established to enable him to manage difficult feelings, to demonstrate a lack of fear, a curiosity, and even a welcoming of the potentially destructive parts of himself. Perhaps he would experience these feelings as a crucial communication of what he had experienced and of what he had and could survive.

Dokter et al. (2011, p. 186) suggest that "symbolic play and dramatic representation may support the child to move from 'acting out' to reflection and thought." Lewis et al. (2000, p. 200) point out that "people do not learn emotional modulation as they do geometry or the names of state capitals." They learn it implicitly from "the presence of an adept external modulator" (Dales & Jerry, 2008, p. 283; Wilkinson, 2010). The role of the therapist as player, facilitator, and modulator seemed crucial to the emerging themes of Jonah's play. Attachment theory tells us that attunement and reciprocity are significant qualities of bonding that reflect mutual awareness and create emotional resonance. For the child who has experienced a disrupted attachment to have this modelled in the therapeutic relationship is inherently healing. Good secure attachment is playful and creates a neurochemistry of bonding (Cozolino, 2002). It seems crucial that in trauma-based dramatherapy, the therapist can play alongside the child and facilitate and contain the experience of the child's play effectively.

An infant between 3 and 6 months of age mainly uses sight and sound to gauge their parents' emotional responses. Positive attunement creates reciprocal joy and delight, creating emotional resonance (Schore, 2013). In relationships in which there is a lack of positive resonance, the child learns to avoid the parent's gaze, experiencing it as confirmation of their unworthiness in receiving and being loved. Jonah told me that the black toy mermaid's eyes were to be avoided, by all means, as it meant that children *'lost their hearts and died inside'*. In the first session, Jonah had told me that he did not have a heart, then of puppet Jonah's heart being attacked by the knight. Between this and Jonah's following session, his mother reported that Jonah had appeared more distressed in his behaviour. We talked about how he might be feeling dysregulated and unsure of the role of mother and what it meant. Collins (2020) writes of how exhausting new learning can be as children's brains actively install new learning and prune synaptic connections no longer as useful to them.

Having his mother in his sessions was fundamental to this therapy, so she witnessed the therapeutic relationship developing and could mirror the core components when Jonah invited her to play. I had felt and modelled empathy for Jonah and the characters' dilemmas. I gently encouraged engagement in the creative process to support Jonah to find creative and spontaneous solutions to the unfolding drama. By engaging in the play narrative, I had come to know Jonah and facilitated his capacity to discover himself.

Jonah's story served as a conversation between us, allowing us to explore and deepen our experience of his metaphors and internal world. The conversation allowed for increased empathy and curiosity and supported Jonah to create a more coherent narrative for the characters. Even when the characters were sleeping, Jonah reflected that they were '*too tired to play the good and bad fight*'. Hughes (2017) calls these kinds of conversations affective-reflective dialogues and maintains that they are fundamental to therapy with abused and neglected children. Jonah's metaphorical narrative enabled him to develop a language to explain feelings, thoughts, and behaviour. Having a violent and abusive father would have impacted Jonah's internal world. Field (1997) argues that infants and toddlers have little capacity to understand the nature of cruelty and neglect, but they are strongly influenced by trauma and by physical and emotional una-vailability of their primary carers. Jonah had had no foster father to balance out this initial imprint, and in his therapy, he was unable to fathom, even in play, how to manage this relationship.

Outcomes

The following week, Jonah's adoptive mother reported that he had been '*like a different child*'. He seemed less angry, less manic in activity, and more relaxed. It seemed that his work in therapy had enabled a change that he was able to take into his everyday life.

Jonah's experiences of being held and experiencing reciprocal delight in relationship with his mother seemed to have an impact on his characters to whom he allowed an expanded range of affect.

Jonah and I played a game at my therapy window called the 'boomerang heart'. Jonah would physically throw away his imaginary heart and we would imagine it boomeranging back to him. '*Ha*', I would exclaim, '*it's landed on your elbow, or your toes, or your tummy*'. Jonah firmly said 'no' to all of these. After several turns, Jonah turned to me and said, '*I know where it is Sarah*', as he pointed to his heart space on his chest and proudly announced '*here*'. When I asked how it felt, he said, '*Okay*' and then told me that he loved his adopted grandad, and mum and dad.

Several months later, Jonah walked into his session and proudly told me: '*I have a heart now, Sarah, because I have found someone to love*'. He pointed at his mother.

Acknowledgements

I would like to add my great appreciation to Jonah's family and to Jonah, without whom this chapter would not have been possible.

My special thanks go to Dr Phil Jones and Madeline Andersen-Warren for their continued support and encouragement of my writing.

References

Bowlby, J. (1982). *Attachment and loss* (2nd ed.). Basic Books.

Carey, M. (2017). From implicit experience to explicit story. In M. N. Beaudoin & J. Duvall (Eds.), *Collaborative therapy and neurobiology. Evolving practices in action* (pp. 41–45). Routledge.

Collins, A. (2020). *The music advantage.* Allen & Unwin.

Cozolino, L. (2002). *The neuroscience of psychotherapy: Building and rebuilding the human brain.* W.W. Norton.

Cozolino, L. (2006). *The neuroscience of human relationships: Attachment and the developing social brain.* W. W. Norton.

Cozolino, L. (2017). *The neuroscience of psychotherapy: Healing the social brain.* W. W. Norton.

Crenshaw, D. (2014). Play therapy approaches to attachment issues. In C. Malchiodi & D. Crenshaw (Eds.), *Creative arts and play therapy for attachment problems* (pp. 5–19). Guildford Press.

Dales, J., & Jerry, P. (2008). Attachment, affect regulation and mutual synchrony in adult psychotherapy. *American Journal of Psychotherapy, 62*(3), 283–312.

Dana, D. (2018). *The polyvagal theory in therapy. Engaging the rhythm of regulation.* W. W. Norton.

Dokter, D., Holloway, P., & Seebohm, H. (2011). Playing with Thanatos: Bringing creativity to destructiveness. In D. Doktor, P. Holloway, & H. Seebohm (Eds.), *Dramatherapy and destructiveness. Creating the evidence base, playing with Thanatos* (1st ed., pp. 179–193). Routledge.

Emunah, R. (1994). *Acting for real: Drama therapy process, technique, and performance.* Routledge.

Fahlberg, V. (1991). *A child's journey through placement.* Perspective Press.

Field, T. (1997). The effects of mother's physical and emotional unavailability on emotional regulation: Monographs of the society for research in child development. In F. Putnam (Ed.), *Dissociation in children and adolescents. A developmental perspective* (pp. 208–227). The Guildford Press.

Fonagy, P., Gergely, G., Jurist, E., & Target, M. (2004). *Affect regulation, mentalization and the development of the self.* Karnac.

Gersie, A. (1992). *Earthtales, storytelling in times of change.* Green Print.

Haythorne, D., Crockford, S., & Godfrey, E. (2012). Roundabout and the development of PSYCHLOPS kids evaluation. Chp. 18. In L. Leigh, I. Gersch, A. Dix, & D. Haythorne (Eds.), *Dramatherapy with children, young people and schools: Enabling creativity, sociability, communication and learning.* Routledge.

Howe, D. (2005). *Child abuse and neglect: Attachment, development and intervention.* Palgrave Macmillan.

Hughes, D. (2017). *Building the bonds of attachment: Awakening love in deeply traumatized children* (3rd ed.). Roman & Littlefield.

Irwin, E. (2005). Facilitating play with non-players. A developmental perspective. In A. Weber & C. Haen (Eds.), *Clinical applications of drama therapy* (pp. 3–24). Brunner and Routledge.

Jennings, S. (2011). *Healthy attachments and neuro-dramatic play*. JKP.

Johnson, D. (2000). Developmental transformations: Towards the body as presence. In P. Lewis & D. Johnson (Eds.), *Current approaches in drama therapy* (pp. 87–110). Charles C. Thomas.

Jones, P. (2007). *Drama as therapy: Theory, practice and research* (2nd ed.). Routledge.

Lewis, T., Amini, F., & Lannon, R. (2000). *A general theory of love*. Vintage Books.

Mann Shaw, S. (2016). Stevie and the little dinosaur. A story of assessment in dramatherapy. In S. Jennings & C. Holmewood (Eds.), *International handbook of dramatherapy* (pp. 230–239). Routledge.

Perry, B. (2009). *Examining child maltreatment through a neurodevelopmental lens: Clinical emotions*. Oxford University Press.

Rizzolatti, G., & Sinigaglia, C. (2008). *Mirrors in the brain: How our minds share actions and emotions* (F. Anderson, Trans.). Oxford University Press.

Schore, A. (2013). Relational trauma, brain development and dissociation. In J. Ford & C. Courtois (Eds.), *Treating complex traumatic stress disorder in children and adolescents* (pp. 3-23). Guildford Press.

Siegel, D. (2001). Towards an interpersonal neurobiology of the developing mind: Attachment relationships, 'mindsight', and neural integration. *Infant Mental Health Journal, 22*(1–2), 67–94.

Van der Kolk, B. (2005). Developmental trauma disorder: A new rational diagnosis for children with complex trauma disorders. *Psychiatric Annals, 35*(5), 401–408.

Van der Kolk, B. (2014). *The body keeps the score: Brain, mind, body in the healing of trauma*. Viking.

Wilkinson, M. (2010). *Changing minds in therapy*. W. W. Norton.

Winnicott, D. (2005). *Playing and reality*. Routledge.

3 Narradrama as a Three Act Play

Transformation, neurobiology, and discovery

Pamela Dunne and Renda Dionne Madrigal

Narradrama as a Three Act Play (NTAP) is a subset of Narradrama, which integrates drama therapy, narrative, and the creative arts. In the NTAP process, each participant develops a creative script that explores personal issues through the creation of preferred roles, alternative stories, and preferred outcomes. NTAP offers a unique approach to the development of a preferred role and includes a creative workbook documenting the emerging preferred role in the play that parallels personal process. A final performance of the play offers expanded opportunities for self-growth through integration aided by reflective processing and witnessing of new alternative stories. The various aspects of the three-act play directly challenge fixed patterns of behaviour and create neural networks to new ways of being.

Case study utilising narrative research, community-based participatory research, practice-based research, and Narradrama research

Viewing NTAP within an indigenous worldview, the question becomes – whose story serves as the healing modality? Narrative research (NR) makes no claim of "objective knowledge," and invites multiple perspectives (Gaddis, 2004; Tootell, 2004; Moen, 2006). Local knowledge and skills of the participants are welcomed (Beaudoin et al., 2016; Redstone, 2004; Epston, 2001; Dulwich Centre Publications, 2004).

Community-based participatory research (CBPR) is a significant advance in research with American Indian/Alaska Native and other historically marginalised communities. The guiding principle in CBPR involves co-learning, bringing community and researchers together to promote community empowerment and agency (Gray et al., 2010; Cornwall & Jewkes, 1995).

Practice-based research (PBR) (Miller, 2014, 2017) takes account of the subjective experience of the participants and considers important elements such as social, cultural, and geographical factors with diverse populations. Treatments found effective by local communities or specific ethnic groups are welcomed. This person-centred approach follows an individualised arts-based method to assessment/research.

DOI: 10.4324/9781003082897-7

What we take, however, from these approaches must be placed within an oral history perspective, for ancestral stories of being are the indigenous people's oral history. It is the story contained within the words that carries forward who the indigenous people are and the wisdom and strength to face adversity at the present time. Oral history, through a post-modern approach (Beard, 2017) serves as an "example of historical narrative-making that treats individual testimonies as mediated cultural processes rather than direct experience" (p. 529). In essence, within an NTAP view, ancestral stories and roles created from them contain the 'medicinal' tools needed for healing today.

A Narradrama inquiry (Savage, 2016) with adolescents who developed animated versions of a personal public service announcement (PPSA) indicated how the Narradrama process could benefit the final development of the PPSA performances and self-identity of adolescents.

This study integrated NR, CBPR, and PBR. A co-research approach facilitates co-learning involving collaboration between the researcher and the participants and is documented through interviews, journal entries, stories, collage, and maps. Through this process meaning emerges. A definitional ceremony involving the retelling and telling of stories utilises group participants acting as witnesses and reflectors. Incorporating definitional ceremony within a therapeutic process has been shown to open opportunities for participants to discover personal strengths and revise their identity (Cao, 2020; Leahy et al., 2012; Speedy et al., 2004). With NTAP, participants created a preferred role, story, and preferred outcome, drawing on wisdom gained from ancient stories, which they crafted into a three-act play.

The research question was whether participants in the NTAP process would develop new insights (wisdom) useful for their life. At the beginning of the group, members were asked a question: *What kind of wisdom are you hoping to gain from the process?*

At the end of the NTAP process participants, costumed in their preferred role, participated in a modified talking circle in which they responded to narrative questions from the point of view of their preferred roles. Definitional ceremony aspects of the telling and retelling of stories through verbal response, art and movement occurred with participants as witnesses and reflectors. A summary focused on commonalities in strengths gained, wisdom gained, and impactful components of the NTAP. Members presented a representation of the most transformative and impactful moments in art, poetry, song, or journal entry. These selections were developed into a pictogram, and video art form. The video art piece was displayed on the internet as a healing offering for the community, expanding as community members responded back to NTAP participants via a Zoom chat box.

NTAP group

The 11 participants represented a wide age range up to 70. Seven participants were adults and four were teenagers. Gender was evenly divided. The group contained eight American Indian, two Caucasian, and one Hispanic group members. The group ran for two hours weekly over eight weeks, with a ninth community performance and the Zoom chat box.

Zoom and the pandemic

Prior to the pandemic, our work included a combination of both live and virtual (Zoom) participants, all engaged in action together. We were familiar with the online Zoom medium and pushed ourselves to become even more creative. For NTAP, large group and break out rooms were utilised for art, animation, video, whiteboard community art, and performance. Individual participant screens transformed into stages for puppet shows or live performances. Experiencing the effects of isolation during the pandemic, participants welcomed Zoom to connect, convey their creativity, and express emotions. As facilitators, taking in full body language and subtle expression represented a difficult challenge (especially with large groups), so invitational questions, use of the chat box, and small and large group sharing filled in gaps. Ethical practices around Zoom and confidentiality were additionally disclosed.

Evaluation process

Understanding the viability and usefulness of a Narradrama process within indigenous communities was a focus of the NTAP co-research.

The NTAP project proposed to

1 assess the viability/feasibility and helpfulness of the process for a mixed group, primarily American Indian/Alaska Native group participants.
2 assess and describe the strengths gained from the process from the perspective of a preferred role.

Philosophical and theoretical framework of NTAP

The foundation of Narradrama is narrative therapy, with principles and research from interpersonal neurobiology and positive psychology. Narradrama is grounded in a humanistic belief that we all possess the propensity for positive change and agency in our own healing. Positive emotions have a 'broadening effect' on the momentary thought-action repertoire. They allow us to discard automatic responses and instead look for creative, flexible, and unpredictable new ways of thinking and acting (Fredrickson, 2004). In NTAP, the therapeutic and creative process contributes to positive well-being, combined with a sense that one's life is good, meaningful, and worthwhile. These are critical components of subjective well-being (Lyubomirsky, 2007).

NTAP group process

NTAP takes place within a collaborative, supportive group process that connects individuals to one another. Participants, as authors of their three-act plays, re-story parts of their history, imagine new possibilities, experience unexpected outcomes, and gain insights into their strengths. Each aspect of play development is explored from a Narradrama perspective, such as preferred roles, scene work, prologue, epilogue, play structure, stage design, staging, reflection, and interpersonal connection to team members. Group members, through scaffolding techniques, reflect on previous work and integrate new preferred roles as well as witnessing and honouring others. Participants receive weekly workbook pages designed to generate a deeper exploration of the roles, themes, and encounters in the play as well as opportunities to grow personally in understanding themselves and their preferred futures. Reflective processes include the telling and retelling of stories. The process culminates in a live performance.

The three acts of NTAP

The three acts follow specific NTAP processes, creative workbook exercises, and play development. Within these acts, neuroscience, narrative and positive psychology principles, reflective questions, case studies, and examples are highlighted.

Act I

Act I of the NTAP process begins with the introduction of novelty. Group members are invited to co-create an environment using imaginative objects, fabrics, art materials, and other resources in the room, with the spirit of curiosity and play; attuning to each other and themselves thus increasing relational engagement; and igniting curiosity and interest. Neurobiology research suggests that novelty triggers curiosity and a release of dopamine in the brain, a neurotransmitter associated with positive experiences (Chermahini & Hommel, 2010, p. 458; Lhommee et al., 2014, p. 1). Siegel (2014) states that "the playfulness and humour that emerge from the creation of new combinations of things are essential to keep our lives full of vitality" (p. 10).

The warm-ups build a safe, creative, and thriving environment. Participants partner up for mirroring exercises and take turns as leader and follower in exploring their movement preferences and emotions connected with these preferences. Partners co-create a dance revealing their shared movement preferences. Mirroring activates both the sympathetic and parasympathetic nervous systems. It creates the conditions of both safety, which is soothing to the nervous system, and stimulation regulated by the vagal nerve as confirmed in polyvagal theory (Porges, 2011). The social engagement that happens during mirroring allows the mind and body to be both relaxed and energised. In this state there is a creative flow. New information can enter and be integrated.

"Research in neuroplasticity shows us that our brains are continually altering. There is potential to change in a positive direction toward increased calm, compassion, resilience, and vitality" (Goldstein, 2017, p. 338). This is critical for the emergence of preferred identity states.

Moving in ways we prefer changes our world and our place in it, particularly when repetition is used. Repeating and expanding preferred movements aids in repeating experiences connected to positive emotions leading to the possibility of increased synaptic connections (Siegel, 2011; Beaudoin & Zimmerman, 2011). Repetition is also important for strengthening new identity states. "Developing practices and habits, combined with the experience of inhabiting new identity states, corresponds to the strengthening of new neural connections" (Ewing et al., 2017, p. 97).

Participants mindfully reflect in their creative workbooks and share with the group, in a further integrative experience, as they respond to questions about ways of moving that give joy, peace or energy; and questions about preferred aspects of personal identity which became clearer in these moments. The importance of reflective practices after enactment is confirmed by neuroscience research (Damasio, 1994, 1999; Van der Kolk, 2002a, 2002b) indicating that, for therapeutic benefits to occur, both hemispheres of the brain need to be activated. For populations with limited insight and verbal capacities, a form of reflection through action may be helpful.

In the next part of Act I, participants explore supportive roles through distancing or in a more direct way. *Pictorial Theatre*, a playful, distanced approach invites participants to choose from a list of theatre roles (e.g. actor, director, stage manager, lighting designer, playwright, audience member) they want to activate. Participants then bring their *Pictorial Theatre* to life in an *Action Sociogram* where they choose group members to sculpt the roles in their theatre, positioned in the same way as their own theatre diagram. Encouraging playfulness through *Pictorial Theatre* creates possibilities for opening new avenues for social engagement according to neuroscience research:

> Playful states involve the social engagement system that reveals the interplay of the open self with the social world. New combinations of neural firing can emerge, new learning can be encoded, and new ways of being in the world of interacting with others can each contribute to the neuroplasticity needed for long lasting change in psychotherapy.
>
> (Chan & Siegel, 2018, p. 57)

NTAP, then focuses on discovery of personal preferred roles. Preferred roles may emerge through any of the following interventions: a collage of preferred roles, a preferred literary or creative role, a role with fairy tale or mythic characteristics crafted into a preferred role, or a preferred role based on an image or a preferred role suggested by objects or masks. Participants gather in small groups to creatively explore preferred roles through sculpts, improvisation, song, short scenes, dialogues, monologues, and stories.

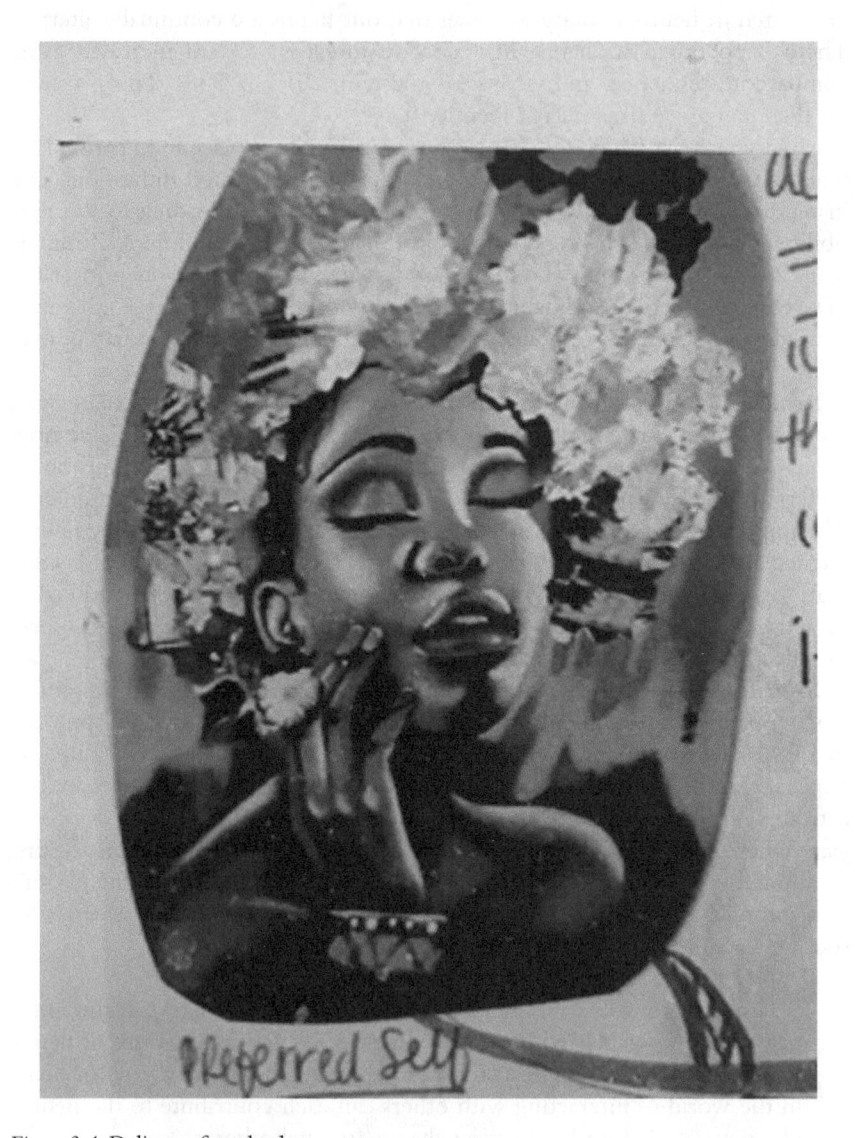

Figure 3.1 Delia: preferred role

Case examples from the NTAP research study Zoom group and the pilot NTAP live group

Delia, an African American woman in her 30s experiencing challenges with depression, created two preferred roles. In Figure 3.1, the first preferred role image (Figure 3.2) Cailtte, emerged to become the protagonist in Delia's play.

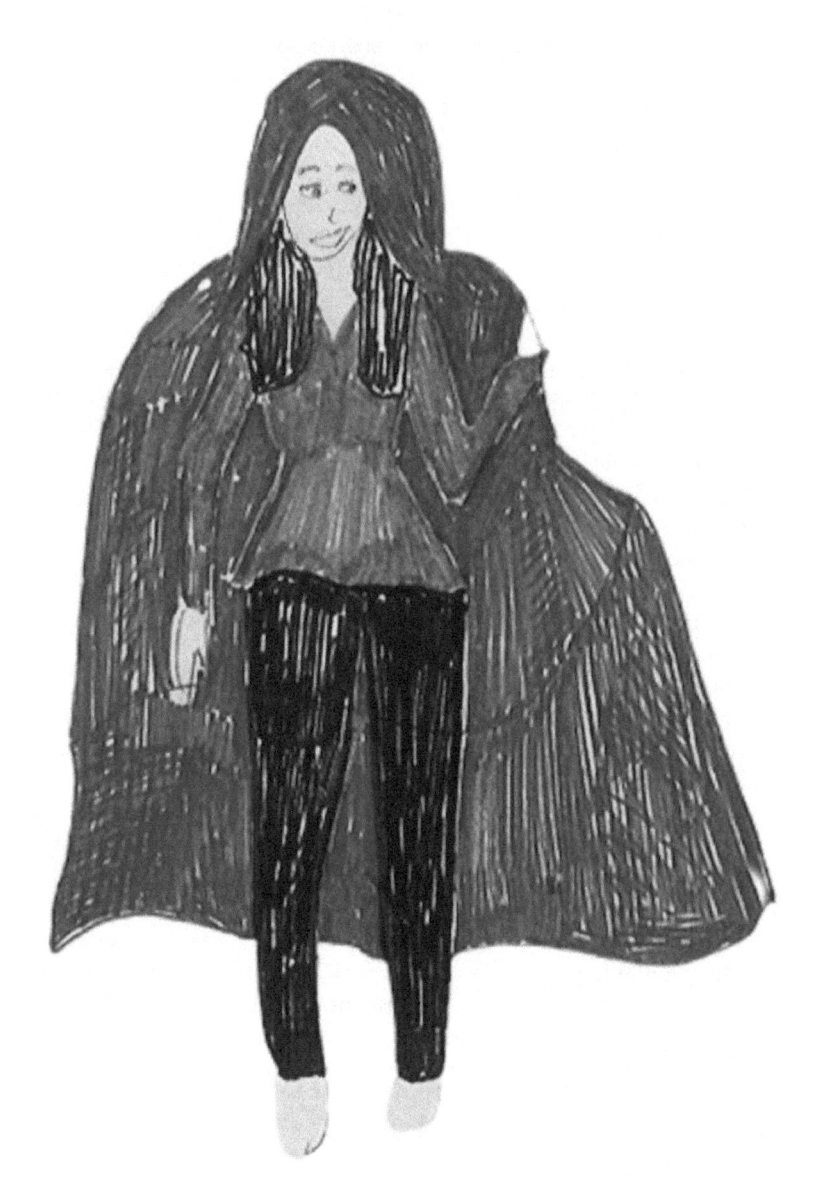

Figure 3.2 Delia: Cailtte

The use of preferred roles is integral in NTAP. By experiencing the actions and physiology of the role, the preferred identity state can be strengthened every time the role is played. Lived associations through the preferred role, "interact with the diverse sensory and cognitive aspects of our lives, creating a coherent set of associations that guide our actions and expectations of the future"

(Ewing et al., 2017, p. 90). In the *Body Keeps the Score*, Van der Kolk described how physically taking on a role in a play changed his son's posture and movement, leading him out of a depressive state in a way that traditional therapy had not been able to do (Van der Kolk, 2014). In order to find our voice we have to be in our bodies – able to breathe fully and able to access our inner sensations (Van der Kolk, 2014). In Somatic Experiencing, this *"resourcing"* puts a person in touch with positive inner feelings of safety, strength, comfort, and optimism, beginning to develop a stable restoration of balance (Payne, 2015).

In moving into scenes for NTAP, participants create a short scene between the preferred role and another character in their play. The personality of the preferred role, even though distanced, reflects the abilities, drives, ideas, passions, preferred identity, and traits of the participant. The participant as director coaches the players to enact the scene, which functions as an audition for the preferred role. After the role audition, each participant reflects mindfully, noticing signs of body physiology and connection to the role. After committing to a preferred role, the participant deeply explores the role through dance/movement, song, improvisation, dialogue, story building, writing a letter in role, and responding to reflective questions. As the role deepens, participants *walk the story landscape* (interacting with the environment of the developing story), creating a *storymap* (non-linear exploration of the story) or by *costuming the role* with preferred fabrics.

In another preferred role audition, Izetta, a 51-year-old Native American female having challenges with anxiety, identified the qualities of passion, intensity, perseverance, and confidence in creating her preferred character Beatrice the Brave (Figure 3.3), a historian.

Participants created one-page scenes between their preferred role and ally. They staged readings of these scenes to explore connections with their reflecting partner; for example, What does my preferred role understand about me that I want to hold onto?

In Izetta's support scene, she chose a support character who acted as a translator guide to provide protection and interpretation in gathering information. In this role of Beatrice, she asked the translator guide to tell her the story of the mountain. He played with her questions, releasing information slowly.

The last part of Act I involves the creation of a prologue for the play which spotlights a historical moment in the life of the participant, paralleling a highlighted moment of the preferred role. A wise character (fantasy or realistic) may emerge to deliver the prologue foretelling some important event or struggle in the play.

Delia's prologue, delivered by the role of the narrator, introduced Cailtte, her preferred role. This prologue sets up the character's challenge which will be explored in Act II.

Narrator: *This is the tale of Cailtte, The Wanderer, Singer of Fire, Master of Self. She was a woman like us, who lived most of her life in a peculiar fog of confusion about the past while trying to remain content in the present. Even the best news came with a persistent fear of something she could never shake or understand.*

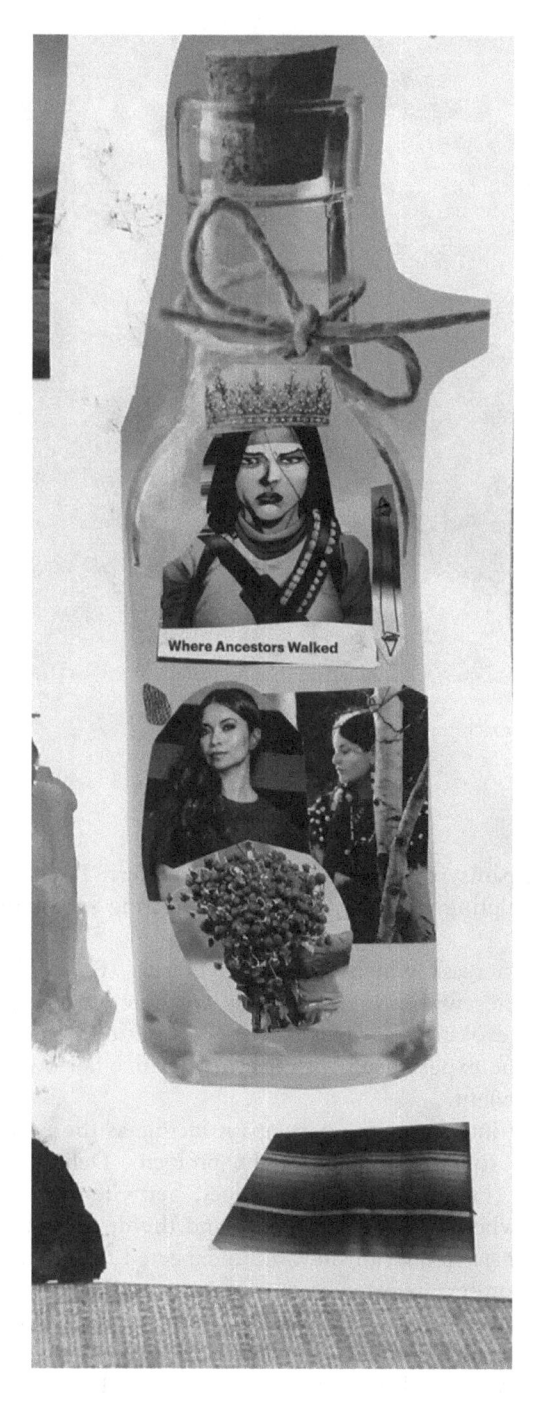

Figure 3.3 Izetta: preferred role *Beatrice the Brave*

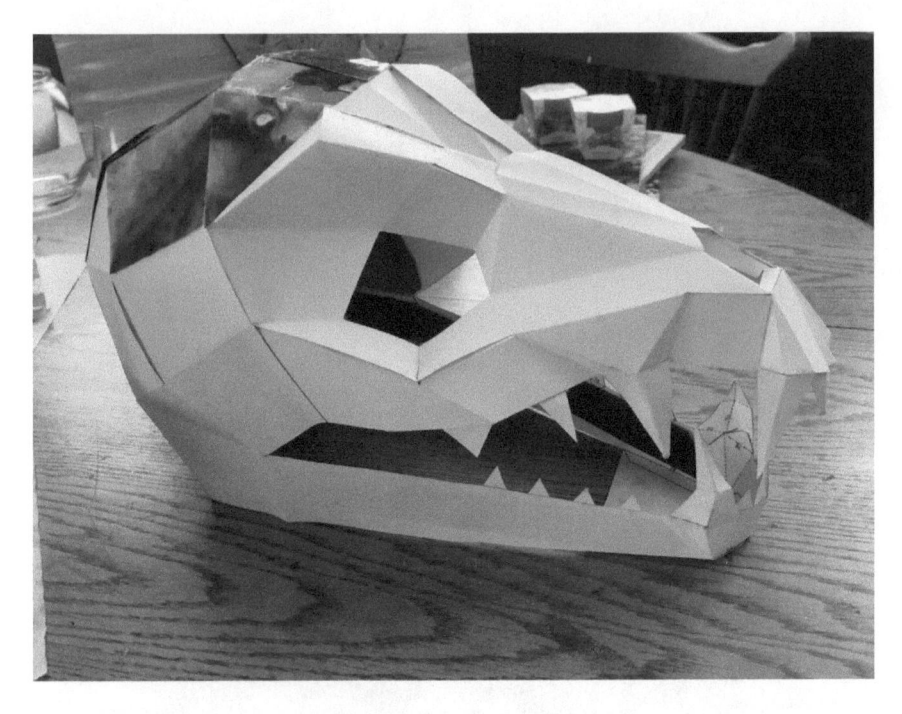

Figure 3.4 Delia: Dorich the antagonist

Act II

In Act II, participants explore challenges of the preferred role through artmaking, drawing, sculpting with clay, painting, or creating a mask of this externalised problem.

Delia created a mask which she named Dorich (Figure 3.4), a demonic antagonist character with a loud booming voice and a looming and formidable body size, evoking fear. This challenged Cailtte (preferred role) to face the temptation she experienced with fear, to sacrifice her own well-being for someone else's benefit.

The facilitator interviews the participant in role as the problem, to determine exceptions to the influence of the problem. Delia created an *image-conflict storyboard* (Figure 3.5), which helped her visualise the conflict, the *darkest moment* (when all hope was gone), and the development of her story. The *image-conflict storyboard* can show an unexpected *twist*, a moment when it seems the protagonist is defeated.

In her *image-conflict storyboard*, Delia showed the middle of the play, starting with protagonist Cailtte and her support Maith travelling to the Guild of Light to ask for help to get back to her own time/realm. They are intercepted by *Dorich*. During the encounter, *Cailtte* drinks a magic potion that she believes

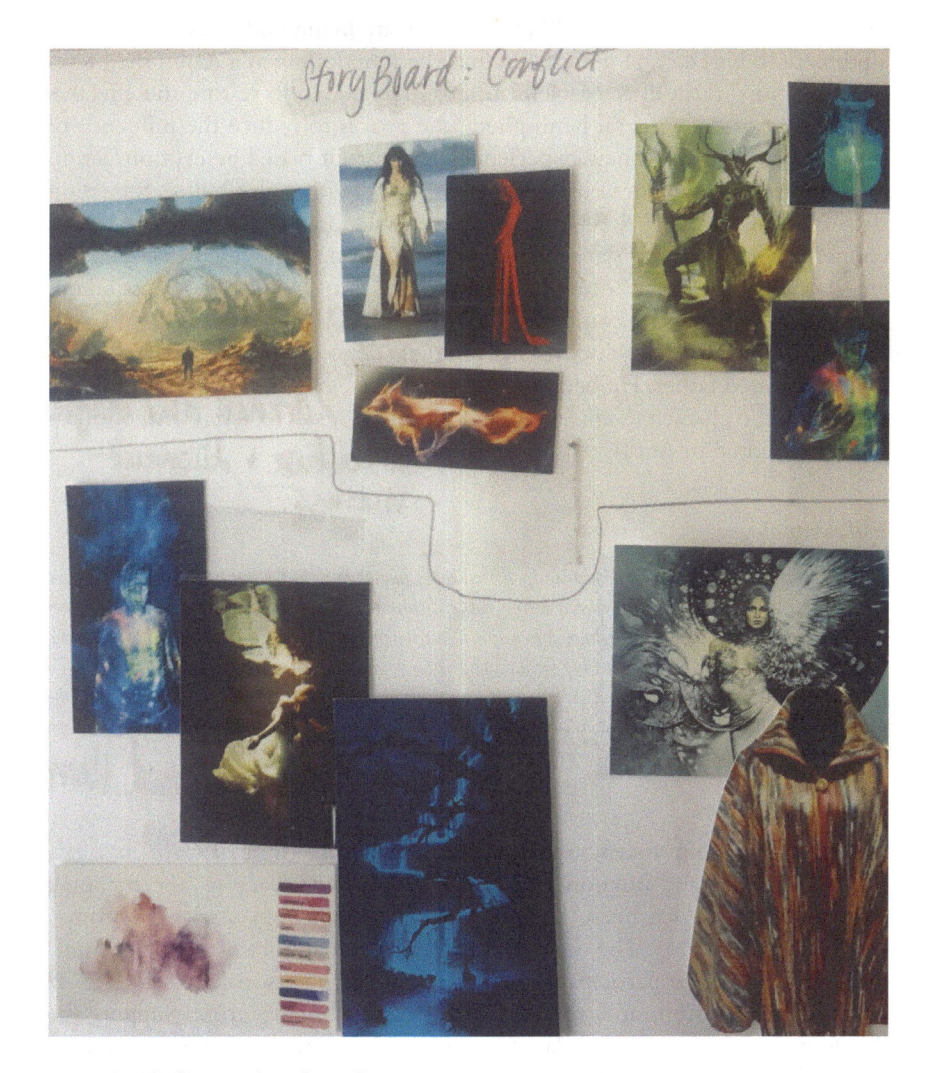

Figure 3.5 Delia: storyboard conflict

will give her extra strength/power, but it impairs her true magical abilities and she falls into a nearby river and is swept away under the water. This *darkest moment* has a *twist*. After falling into the water, Cailtte encounters a hallucination of Foirfe, the Evil Queen, who tempts her to join her dark army. Cailtte transforms the strength of the Evil Queen, into her own positive strength (the *twist*), and refuses to join the dark army.

Externalising masks, *image-conflict storyboards*, and *storymaps* provide distance between the participant and the problem and open space for the participant to make choices congruent with their preferred self and values as shown in

Delia's *image-conflict storyboard*. "When people are living under the influence of a problem, their cerebral hemisphere may be functioning at a diminished level of integration" (Duvall & Maclennan, 2017, p. 19), so to restore the effective functioning of the cerebral hemisphere, the goal is to reduce the influence of the problem. Repeated new experiences will disrupt biased perception/action loops built into problem saturated stories, allowing new possibilities for action (Ewing et al., 2017, pp. 94–95). "Exploring a positive emotion that could counter the problematic state offers a second option from which to contain or eradicate the problem" (Beaudoin, 2017, p. 30). This step into new possibilities is the heart of the rising conflict for NTAP.

Izetta was surprised to discover her prologue delivered by the preferred character's deceased father. He became another ally for the character development, expressing the character's challenge, and serving as a call to action. All of this is further explored in Act II.

Father's prologue

> On my deathbed I told Beatrice (preferred role's name) to fight for the Indians. To never give up, even if she was fighting a losing battle, because it was the only way she could be free. Beatrice was always a fighter, a free spirit, but when she turned thirteen her belief in herself fell away. She began searching for acceptance and validation of her worth from the mainstream world – that was her yardstick, but she could never be mainstream, because it's not who she was. It wasn't until my death that she stopped and looked at who she was and started to get to know that person.

In Act II, the group journeys into a transitional space (liminal space) navigating in uncertain and unknown territory. The liminal space is "the stripping away of what one has been, but not yet arrived at whom one will become" (Volkas, 2016, p. 114). The discovery of the individual stories in this act, parallels discoveries other participants are making through personalised stories. The support, imagination, and co-creation happening in the group support the developing structure of the play. Over time, as positive experiences emerge within the framework of the group, feelings of safety, comfort, and calm help members settle into the group. These experiences can start to become hardwired into our psyche, aided by the positive emotions and the promoting of more positive relationships (Goldstein, 2017, pp. 338–358).

Continuing exploration of important discoveries in the liminal space, group members each participate in co-constructing a *creative toolbox* where they make or collect tools that will help them in confronting obstacles. The toolbox begins filling up with inspiring or energising images, photos, objects, created tools (e.g. imagination enhancers), and mindfulness meditations which move the story forward. Some participants choose to *enchant* a particular tool. Delia's creative toolbox included natural objects like rocks to help ground her preferred role and a *cape of empowerment* dubbed *guild of light* to connect her to

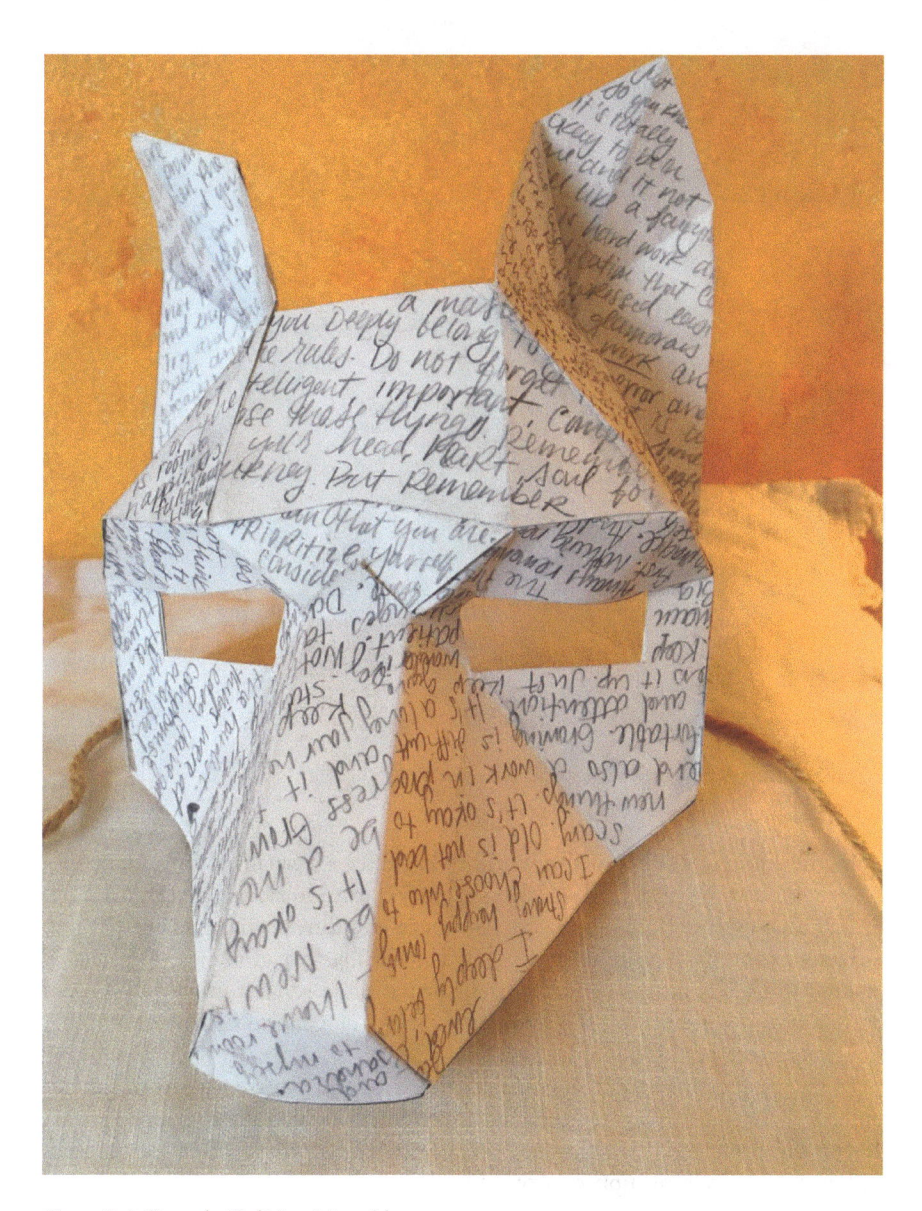

Figure 3.6 Sinnach, Delia's spirit guide

what was essential. A new spirit guide, Sinnach, emerged from her enchanting of the cape.

Delia explored Sinnach as a spirit mask (Figure 3.6) which she created with wisdom phrases gathered from letters she had written to herself. These phrases were written on the mask and internalised by her preferred role.

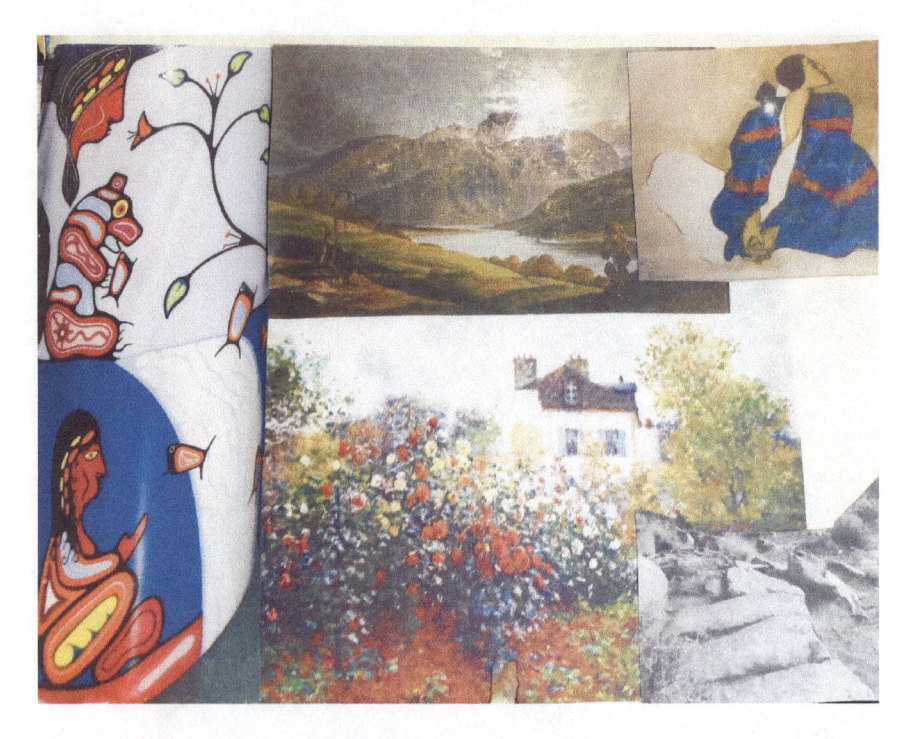

Figure 3.7 Izetta's preferred role Strengths

In the liminal space and the workbook, Izetta externalised important discoveries about the preferred self that she pulled from her heritage (Figure 3.7). Strong images from both her Native American and European heritage emerged.

Izetta's toolbox (Figure 3.8) contained a *lodestone* for guidance, the *stone of destiny* which was necessary for her transformation, a *portal* from which she can draw wisdom and stability, the *red cape* of *strength and protection*, and a *sword* that transforms to a *pen of truth*.

Izetta, used poetry to create an initiation rite as a *transforming ritual* for her preferred character. She then directed a scene in which another group member played the preferred character and recited the poem while other participants gathered in a circle of support around her.

> *I search the world over digging deep into the past*
> *To reveal the voices of yesterday*
> *It's wide the net I cast*
> *I search the world over*
> *Looking here and looking there*
> *The truth of our existence*
> *The past I want laid bare.*

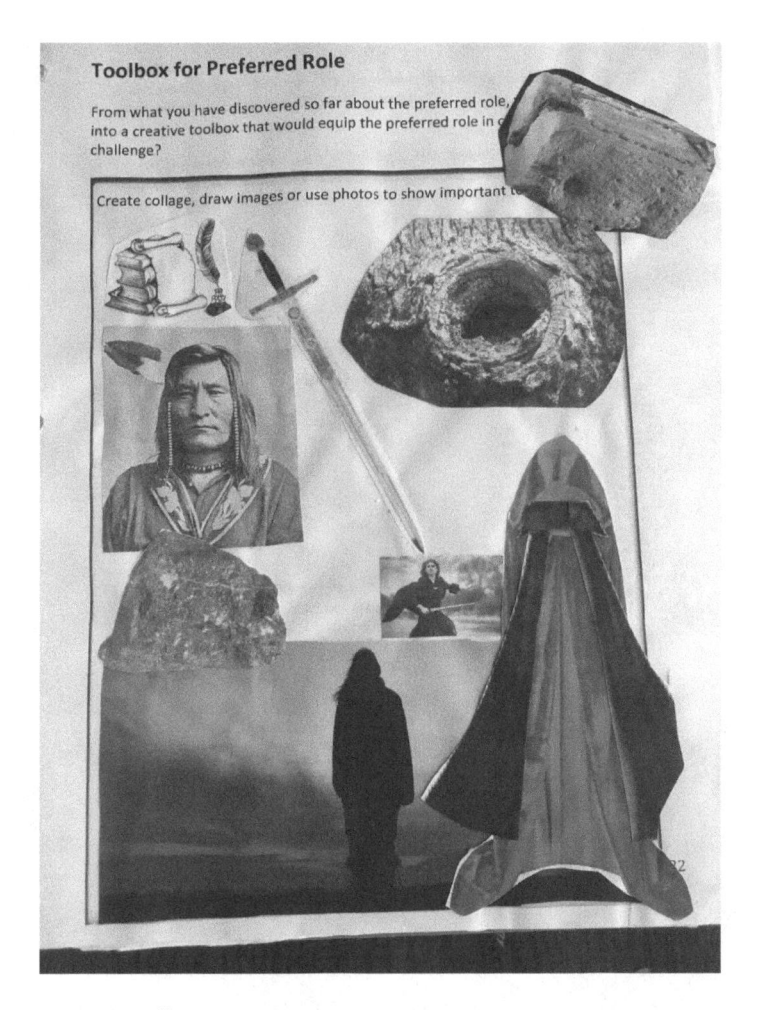

Figure 3.8 Izetta's toolbox

The process of psychotherapy itself often follows an initiation rite structure-embarking on a journey toward change, confronting the unknown and returning to a changed self (Volkas, 2016, p. 115). NTAP reflects this process which includes highly charged emotions, which according to Siegel (2011, p. 85), are "important for structural change in the brain to happen. When we are not engaged emotionally the experience is less memorable and the structure of the brain is less likely to change".

Before their final embarkation on the journey, participants create *enchanted wisdom objects or wisdom masks* to remind them to hold their inner wisdom. The emotional charge of the *enchanted wisdom object* or *wisdom mask* helps the participants in confronting fears and tests. According to Cohen and Findlay

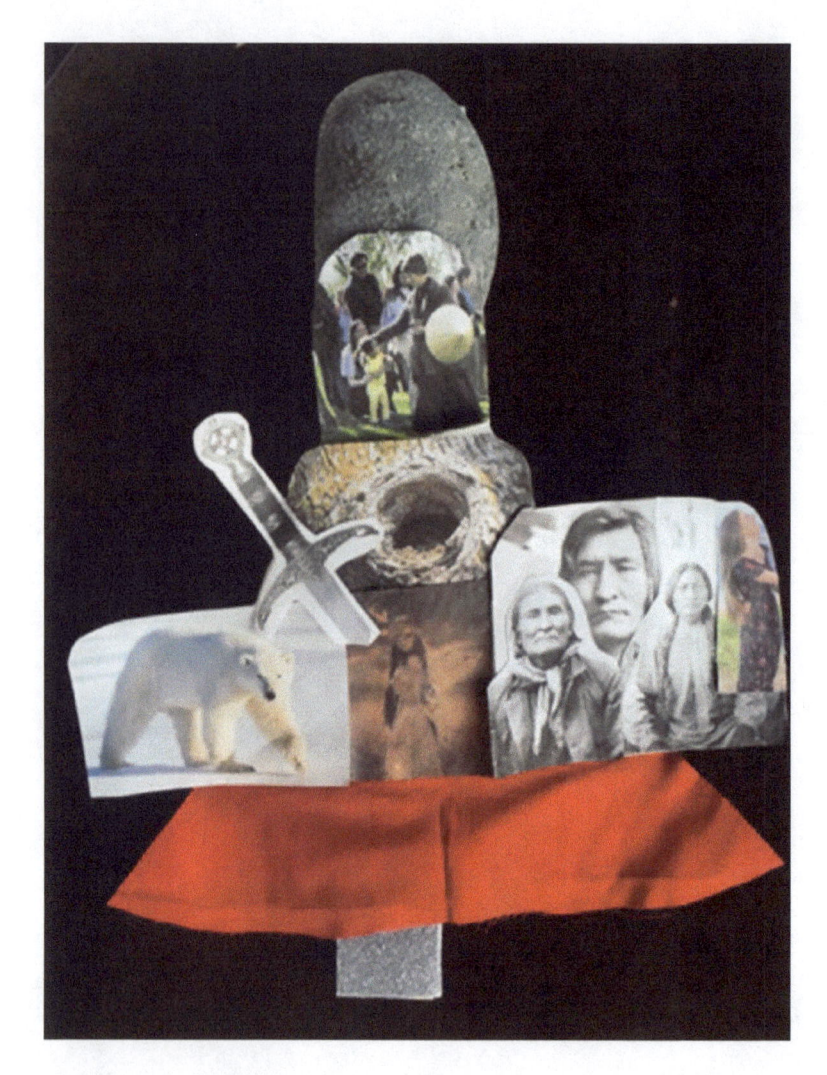

Figure 3.9 Izetta's enchanted pen

(2015, pp. 171–204), the very act of creating the physical object, may directly access the social and emotional self, providing clients with opportunities to process emotions. This provides an entryway into emotional expressivity which according to Siegel (2011, p. 85) makes it possible for the brain structure to change.

For Izetta, the sword from the past became the pen (Figure 3.9) to use to reveal the truth. Through the pen, she expressed her authentic self, connected to confidence and resiliency from which she was able to draw a stable base of strength connected to her ancestors and heritage.

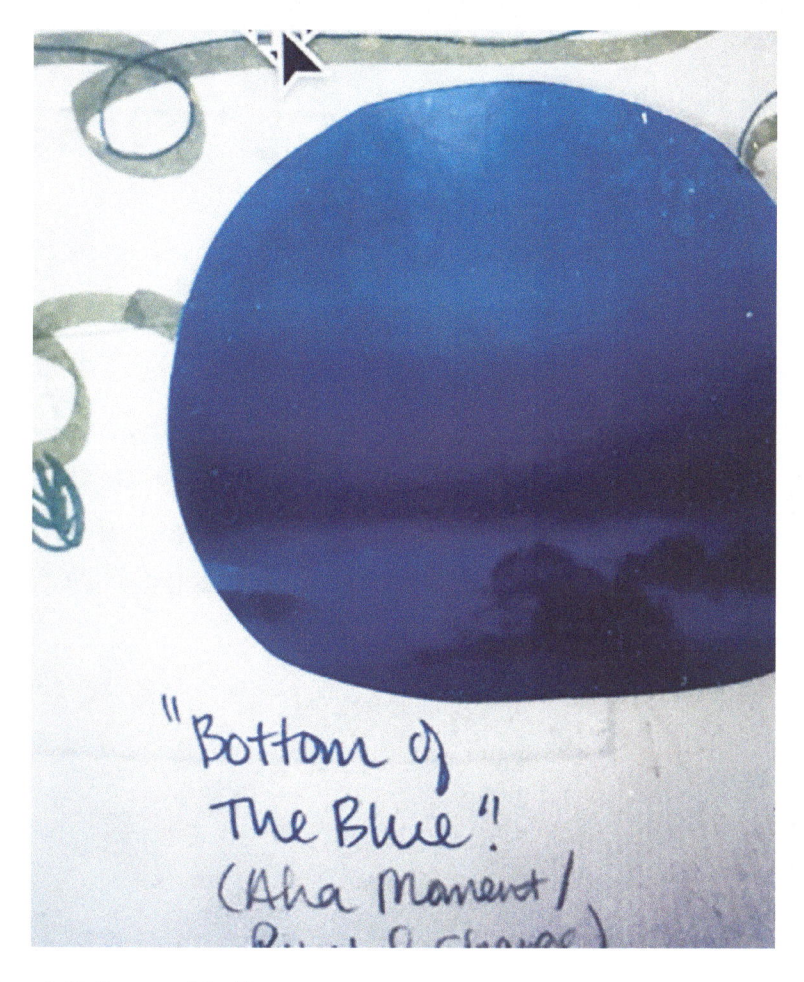

Figure 3.10 Bottom of the blue

In Act II, the plot further develops as new emerging pivotal moments and stories come forth, rich with meaning and possibility. "Rich story development is a key feature of this transitional phase and fertile ground for pivotal moments." Pivotal moments are partially formed, fleeting experiences, vulnerable to disappearance unless acknowledged and anchored in the external world. "They provide a calling, inviting movement toward a reconsideration and reincorporation of identity" (Duvall & MacLennan, 2018, p. 22). These nontraditional, fleeting moments which emerge require an anchoring and recognition as they hold the values and hopes of the participants and their emerging plays.

In a *pivotal moment*, Delia became aware of a transforming image, *bottom of blue* (Figure 3.10). Immersing herself in the blue, she expanded the moment,

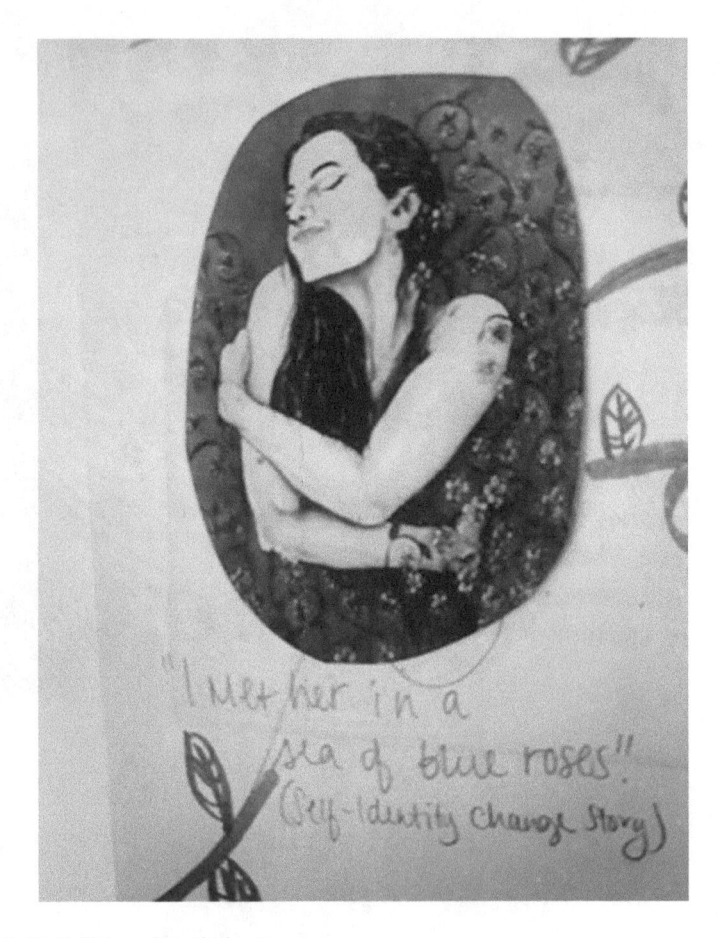

Figure 3.11 Delia's preferred identity

experiencing the richness of it, and reflecting on the meaning. Associations with the colour blue appeared in her developing play, providing support and nurture for her protagonist.

> A story serves as a temporal map, providing space over time to alleviate the problematic effects of life's distressful transitions on people's experience of identity and agency.
>
> (Duvall & Beres, 2011, p. 15)

Delia constructed the fantasised journey of her preferred role, Cailtte, becoming aware of her changed preferred identity through the image "I Met Her in a Sea of Blue Roses" (Figure 3.11). She expanded this image in the play as a poem about the protagonist floating down the river into the *loch of light*.

Dissent (excerpt)
Melt and Meld. Her fear melts down, away.
Escape from her body.
Her skin weighty, simple.
Places unknown, impossible.
Downstream, Plunged below, Swiftly guiding.
Babbles and batters.
She floats to the end of the river.
Graceful for a moment.
Swept down beneath the glassy surface.
Sinking.
Deeper.
Deeper
Panic . . . swim . . . reach.
Strange and Familiar.

In Act 11, alongside the personal group process, plays move forward paralleling the journey of the preferred role in critical development scenes which forward the plot. Other developed scenes focus on setbacks and how the preferred role strategises using their tools, wisdom object/mask, and ally to move past the setback. Discovery scenes focus on clarity of vision, values, and ways to defeat the obstacle.

Act III

Entering NTAP, Act III, participants continue to integrate values and skills with new learning that has simultaneously occurred with their preferred role in the play development.

"Weaving preferred values and hopeful memories into the problem story, may supplement the fabricating function of the left hemisphere and 're-present' previously implicit, but now explicit, experience back to the right hemisphere with integration into the life story. This new narrative – by combining the sequential, logical, semantic capacity of the left hemisphere with the holistic, emotional, episodic memory of the right hemisphere can be a powerful agent of neural, personal and interpersonal integration" (Siegel, 2012; Duvall & MacLennan, 2018, p. 25, citing Cozolino 2014). In addition, this weaving allows for the experience of *Emodiversity*, or experiencing positive and negative affect independently, which is associated with a self-aware and authentic life, and linked to health and well-being (Schutte et al., 2007; Wood et al., 2008).

Participants looking toward their preferred futures write the last scenes of their play while responding to reflective questions and art interventions. For Izetta this led to the need for a *Community of Cultural Rebels* (Figure 3.12) to engage in activities that help the world by carrying the wisdom of the past forward, leaving little room to be immobilised by anxiety and isolation.

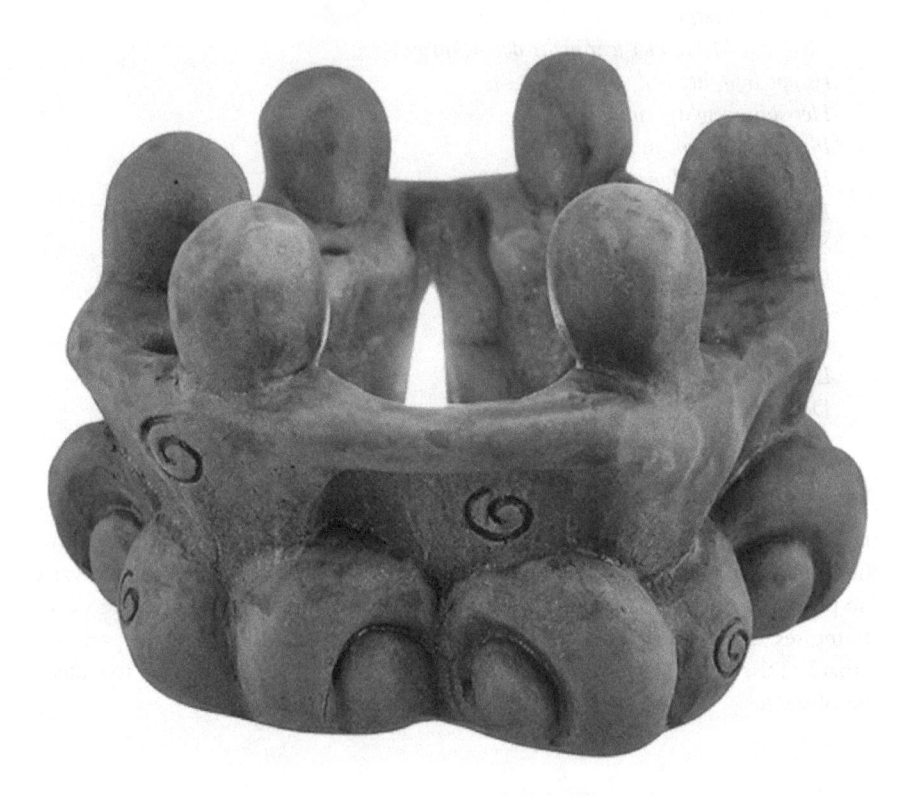

Figure 3.12 Future vision Izetta – *Community of Cultural Rebels*

Delia immersed herself in her future vision with images aiming to integrate inner peace, inner balance, internal shared authenticity with self and others, visibility, grounded, centred, and mindful. In this future she describes herself as having a "voice that is unshakeable" (Figure 3.13).

Participants continue to reflect on their future vision as they complete and present their plays with the whole group acting as reflectors through movement and/or verbal reflection. Participants also consider invitational questions which are grounded in competency. For example, In Act III, questions are posed: What stands out to you as the clearest and most important part of your future vision? What hope becomes more visible?

Some of the plays conclude with an epilogue which brings perspective to the play and closure to the work, while others end in poetry or a climactic moment. Delia performed a journey movement piece interwoven with mythical, poetic scenes depicting a struggle and breaking free to find that, in the end, what she was looking for was herself. For Izetta a con artist character emerged from a character collage. She expanded this through embodiment to explore a role she was resisting, which became a key element in her transformation.

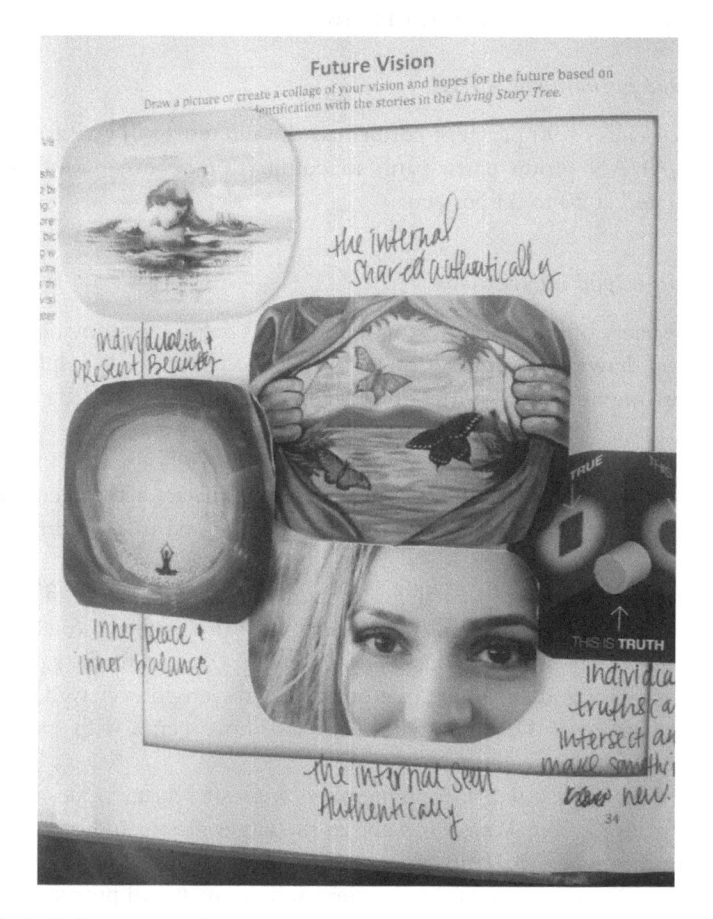

Figure 3.13 Delia's future vision

Rehearsal, performance, witnessing, and reflections

The ultimate performance is a culmination of parallel process, refining scenes and themes and honouring new identities and clarity of future vision. The distancing the preferred role provides opens a window for the participant to see their process unfold. During the performance, the audience is not only viewing a work of art unfolding before them but also being witness to a transformation. "There is an inherent connectedness between the audience and the performer wherein support of the performer's courage, openness, and journey begins before the first line of her script" (Dunne, 2016, p. 152).

Reflections, either individual or as a reflecting team are a key part of the NTAP process. With public performances, individual audience members may perform a one-minute reflection as silent witnesses. Participants act as reflectors to each performance viewed.

Outcomes of the NTAP Oral History Project

Viability and feasibility of NTAP

Attendance rates of 90 per cent confirmed the interest of NTAP for a mixed group of AI/AN group participants in comparison to other kinds of programmes rated at 20 to 33 per cent.

NTAP most helpful interventions

Having a variety of interventions was identified as helpful for moving the story forward and drawing wisdom. A list of NTAP modalities most helpful to participants in moving their stories forward in positive directions included the following:

> *Landscape maps:* Maps of the land the preferred character travelled through, showing strengths gained or obstacles encountered to overcome in each land.
>
> *Preferred role monologues:* Participants came dressed in role and delivered monologues written from the perspective of the preferred role.
>
> *Preferred role, ally,* and *externalised problem masks:* Created masks gave further role insights and expanded role qualities and were interviewed.
>
> *Preferred role scenes:* Dialogue with allies and short scenes with special tools were written.
>
> *NTAP witnessing practices:* Group members witnessed monologues, scenes, or art forms in a breakout room and in the larger group, and offered reflections through verbal, movement, gesture, or art.
>
> *Storymaps:* Non-linear maps show story development and progression.
>
> *Creative toolbox:* Included helpful tools for the preferred roles, some of which were enchanted.
>
> *Song making:* Identified or created songs which participants resonated with as a resource.
>
> *Character collage:* A collage of images, colours, and shapes reflecting traits of the preferred roles or other roles.

When the preferred character was asked, "What part of the NTAP process was most helpful in uncovering wisdom?" Mark responded, "Part of the uncovering of things that led to wisdom is best reflected by hearing other people's struggles and realising that we are all in this human condition. This thinking makes us stronger and this was the greatest wisdom."

Mary said, "The *storymap* helped me develop my story and the impact of how we relate to each other."

Ryan stated, "*The character collages* and the *storymaps* were really helpful."

NTAP witnessing practices resonated positively with most members.

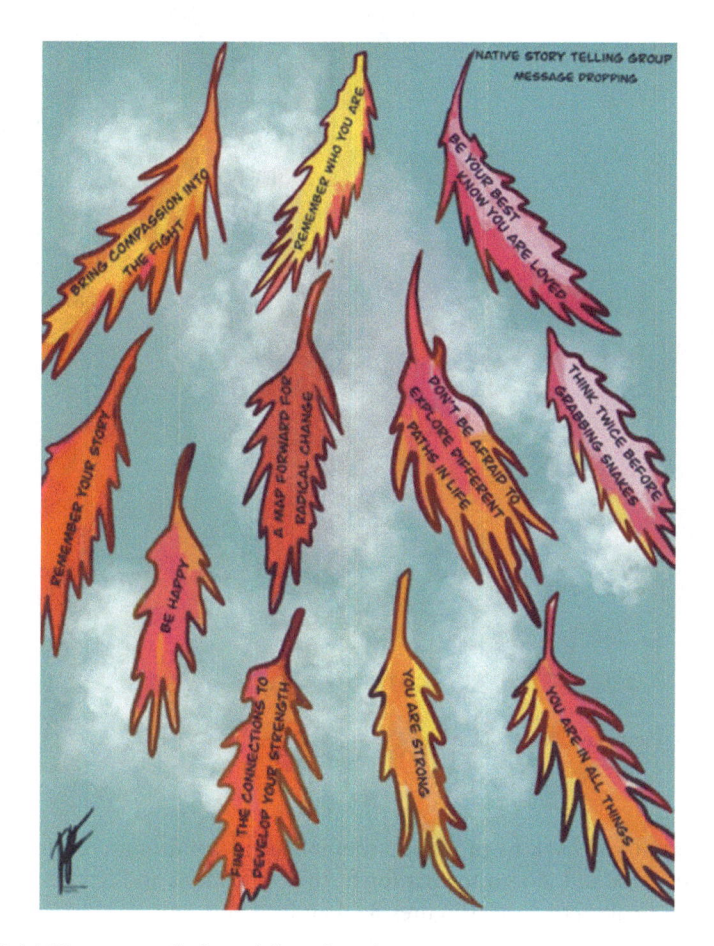

Figure 3.14 Pictogram – feather wisdom droppings

Strengths gained from the perspective of preferred role

Participants began the NTAP group exploring loss and difficulty in their lives. They were asked initially, "If this was a process where you could gain wisdom, what kind of wisdom would you be seeking to gain?" At the conclusion of the groups, participants were asked about wisdom gained from both the perspective of preferred roles and as themselves.

Participants' answers were richer in the preferred role than when answering as individuals. One possibility for this difference is the distance a preferred role provides, so participants are less self-conscious, more playful, and can see from a broader perspective.

A group metaphor emerged of a flock of geese containing identified strengths and wisdom within individuals and within the community (Figure 3.15). This

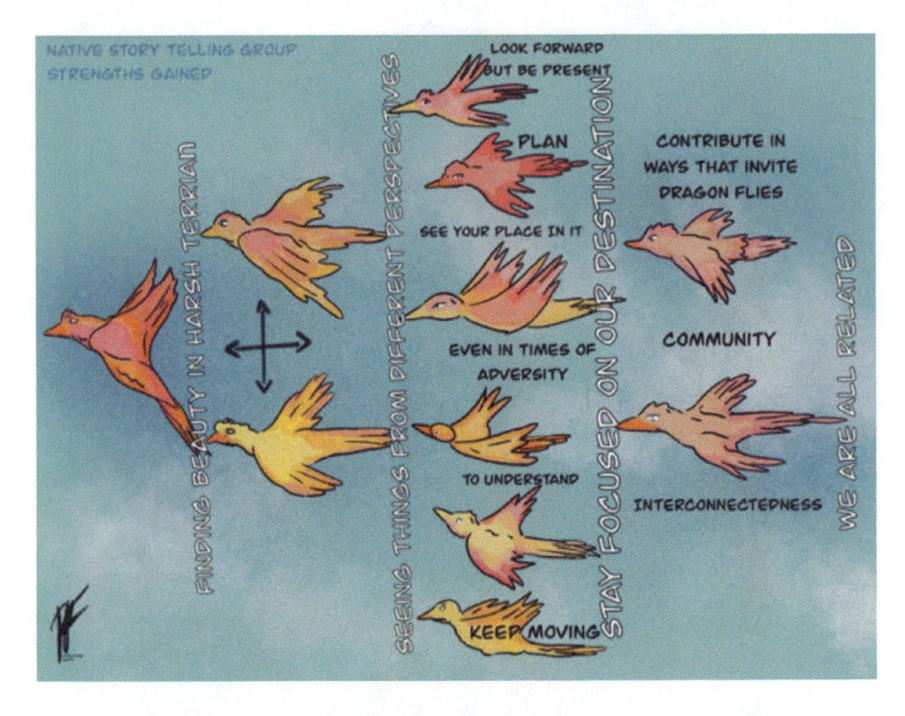

Figure 3.15 Pictogram: flock of strengths

theme was played back to the group members and community online in both a live Facebook and Zoom format for further reflections and feedback and led to the two final pictograms (Figures 3.14 and 3.15).

The community offering of the wisdom video was received and community members reflected in the Zoom chat box. Reflections included, "Amazing! Oh, this creates hope in and of itself, deep bows; How wonderful to pause, to reflect, to listen, to hear."

Promising practices and applications of NTAP

Evaluating a narrative and drama therapy approach using the structure of a three-act play further develops a Narradrama modality and shows the feasibility and strength of this approach for promoting health. Previously, evaluating a process of NTAP had not been applied for viability and meaning-making within indigenous groups. Strengths gained from the perspective of a preferred role were explored through this process. This study helps develop the next steps of NTAP with indigenous populations, aimed at improving the health of tribes and other communities suffering from health disparities and marginalisation.

Acknowledgements

I would like to acknowledge the indigenous people and their supporters for walking on this journey with me through the world of story. None of this would have been possible without you. I would also like to thank Pamela Dunne for her work and relentless dedication to bringing drama and narrative to the world and making it accessible for healing (Renda Dionne Madrigal).

Special thanks for ideas and inspiration from Kamran Afary, Cassandra Ambe, and Betsy Davis; to my husband Mike for his support, patience, kindness, and encouragement in the long writing process; and to Renda Dionne Madrigal for her dedication, compassion, and sensitivity in exploring new ways of accessing the wisdom of ancient stories carried forth to preferred stories and roles with indigenous people (Pamela Dunne).

References

Beard, M. R. (2017). Re-thinking oral history – a study of narrative performance. *Rethinking History*, *21*(4), 529–548. https://doi.org/10.1080/13642529.2017.1333285

Beaudoin, M. N. (2017). Helping clients thrive with positive emotions: Expanding people's repertoire of problem counter-states. In M. Beaudoin & J. Duvall (Eds.), *Collaborative therapy and neurobiology* (pp. 28–39). Routledge.

Beaudoin, M. N., Moersch, M., & Evare, B. (2016). The effectiveness of narrative therapy with children's social and emotional skill development: An empirical study of 813 problem solving stories. *Journal of Systemic Therapies*, *35*(3), 42–59.

Beaudoin, M. N., & Zimmerman, J. (2011). Narrative therapy and interpersonal neurobiology: Revisiting classic practices, developing new emphases. *Journal of Systemic Therapies*, *30*(1), 1–13.

Cao, S. S. (2020). Story variations: Resisting the cultural gaze. *International Journal of Narrative Therapy and Community Work*, *1*, 46–60.

Chan, A., & Siegel, D. (2018). Play and the default mode network: Interpersonal neurobiology, self and creativity. In T. M. Tarlow, T. M. Solomon, & D. Siegel (Eds.), *Play and creativity in psychotherapy* (pp. 39–63). Norton Professional.

Chermahini, S. A., & Hommel, B. (2010). The (b)link between creativity and dopamine: Spontaneous eye blink rates predict and dissociate divergent and convergent thinking. *Cognition*, *115*(3), 458–465.

Cohen, N. H., & Findlay, J. C. (2015). *Art therapy and the neuroscience of relationships, creativity and resiliency*. W. W. Norton.

Cornwall, A., & Jewkes, R. (1995). What is participatory research? *Social Science & Medicine*, *41*, 1667–1676.

Cozolino, L. (2014). *The neuroscience of human relationships: Attachment and the developing social brain* (2nd ed.). W.W. Norton.

Damasio, A. R. (1994). *Descartes' error, emotion, reason and the human brain*. Putnam.

Damasio, A. R. (1999). *The feeling of what happens: Body and emotions and the making of consciousness*. Harcourt Brace.

Dulwich Centre Publications. (2004). Narrative therapy and research. *International Journal of Narrative Therapy and Community Work*, *2*, 29–36.

Dunne, P. (2016). Restoried script performance. In D. Johnson, R. Emunah, & P. Pendzik (Eds.), *The self in performance* (pp. 141–154). Palgrave Macmillan.

Duvall, J., & Beres, L. (2011). *Innovations in narrative therapy: Connecting practice training and research*. W. W. Norton.

Duvall, J., & MacLennan, R. (2018). Pivotal moments, therapeutic conversations, and neurobiology: Landscapes of resonance, possibility, and purpose. In M. N. Beaudoin & J. Duvall (Eds.), *Collaborative therapy and neurobiology: Evolving practices in action* (pp. 15–27). Routledge.

Epston, D. (2001). Anthropology, archives, co-research and narrative therapy: An interview with David Epston. In D. Denborough (Ed.), *Family therapy: Exploring the field's past, present and possible futures* (pp. 161–166). Dulwich Centre Publications.

Ewing, J., Estes, R., & Like, B. (2017). Narrative neurotherapy (NNT): Scaffolding identity states. In M. N. Beaudoin & J. Duvall (Eds.), *Collaborative therapy and neurobiology* (pp. 87–99). Routledge.

Fredrickson, B. L. (2004). Gratitude, like other positive emotions, broadens and builds. In R. A. Emmons & M. E. McCullough (Eds.), *Series in affective science. The psychology of gratitude* (pp. 145–166). Oxford University Press. https://doi.org/10.1093/acprof:oso/9780195150100.003.0008

Gaddis, S. (2004). Repositioning traditional research: Centering clients' accounts in the construction of professional therapy knowledges. *International Journal of Narrative Therapy and Community Work, 2*, 37–48.

Goldstein, B. (2017). Cultivating curiosity, creativity, and self-awareness through mindful group therapy for children and adolescents. In T. M. Solomon & D. Siegel (Eds.), *Play and creativity in psychotherapy* (pp. 338–358). W. W. Norton.

Gray, N., Oré de Boehm, C., Farnsworth, A., & Wolf, D. (2010). Integration of creative expression into community-based participatory research and health promotion with native Americans. *Family & Community Health, 33*(3), 186–192.

Leahy, M., O'Dwyer, O., & Ryan, F. (2012). Definitional ceremonies in narrative therapy with adults who stutter. *Journal of Fluency Disorders.* https://doi:10:1016/j.jflidis.2012.03.001

Lhommee, E., Batir, A., Quesada, J. L. Ardouin, C., Fraix, V., Seigneuret, E., Chabardes, S., Benabid, A. L., Pollack, P., & Krack, P. (2014). Dopamine and the biology of creativity: Lessons from Parkinson's disease. *Frontiers in Neurology 5, 55*(11), 1–11.

Lyubomirsky, S. (2007). *The how of happiness: A scientific approach to getting the life you want.* Penguin.

Miller, C. (2014). *Assessment and outcomes in the arts therapies: A person-centred approach* (pp. 15–30). Jessica Kingsley.

Miller, C. (2017). Practice-based evidence: Therapist as researcher, using outcome measures. *Dramatherapy, 38*(1), 4–15. https://doi.org/10.1080/02630672.2017.1288263

Moen, T. (2006). Reflections on the narrative research approach. *International Journal of Qualitative Methodology, 5*(4), 1–10.

Payne, P., Levine, P. A., & Crane-Godreau, M. A. (2015). Somatic experiencing: Using interoception and proprioception as core elements of trauma therapy. *Frontiers in Psychology, 6*, Article 423. Corrigendum.

Porges, S. (2011). *The polyvagal theory.* W. W. Norton.

Redstone, A. (2004). Researching people's experience of narrative therapy: Acknowledging the contribution of the client to what works in counselling conversations. *International Journal of Narrative Therapy and Community Work, 2*, 1–6.

Savage, M. (2016). Listening to the voices of young women adopted from foster care through personal public service announcements. *Drama Therapy Review, 3*(2), 196–208.

Schutte, N. S., Malouff, J. M., Thorsteinsten, B., Bhullar, N., & Rooke, S. (2007). A meta-analytic investigation of the relationship between emotional intelligence and health. *Personality and individual Differences, 42*(6), 921–933. https://doi.org/10.1016/j.paid.2006.09.003

Siegel, D. J. (2011). *Mindsight*. Random House.

Siegel, D. J. (2012). *The developing mind: How relationships and the brain interact to shape who we are. Second edition*. Guilford Press.

Siegel, D. J. (2014). *Brainstorm: The power and purpose of the teenage brain*. Tarcher/Penguin.

Speedy, J., & Thompson, G. (2004). Living a more people life: Definitional ceremony as inquiry into psychotherapy outcomes. *International Journal of Narrative Therapy and Community Work, 3,* 43–53.

Tootell, A. (2004). Decentering research practice. *International Journal of Narrative Therapy and Community Work, 3,* 54–66.

Van der Kolk, B. A. (2014). *The body keeps the score: Brain, mind, and body in the healing of trauma*. Viking.

Van der Kolk, B. A. (2002a). *The assessment and treatment of complex PTSD in trauma, consciousness and the body*. Presented at winter seminars at Harvard medical School, Department of Continuing Education. Google Scholar.

Van der Kolk, B. A. (2002b). *Posttraumatic stress disorder and the nature of trauma*. Presented at winter seminars at Harvard medical School, Department of Continuing Education. Google Scholar.

Volkas, A. (2016). Autobiographical therapeutic performance as individual therapy. In S. Pendzik, R. Emunah & D. R. Johnson (Eds.), *The self in performance, autobiographical, self-revelatory, and autoethnographic forms of therapeutic theatre* (pp. 113–129). Palgrave Macmillan.

Wood, A. M., Linley, P. A., Maltby, J., Baliousis, M., & Joseph, S. (2008). The authentic personality: A theoretical and empirical conceptualization and the development of the authenticity scale. *Personality and Individual Differences, 42*(6), 921–933. https://doi:10.1037/0022-0167.55.3.385

Additional reading

Beaudoin, M. N. (2015). Flourishing with positive emotions: Increasing clients' repertoire of problem counter states. *Journal of Systemic Therapies, 3*(34), 1–13.

Dunne, P. (2006). *The narrative therapist and the arts* (2nd ed.). Possibility Press.

Dunne, P. (2010). Narradrama with marginalized groups: Uncovering strengths, knowledges and possibilities. In E. Leveton (Ed.), *Healing collective trauma: Using sociodrama and drama therapy*. Springer Publishing Company.

Dunne, P. (2017). Insights in positive changes: An exploration between the link between drama therapy and neural networks. In M. N. Beaudoin & J. Duvall (Eds.), *Alternative therapies*. Routledge.

Dunne, P., & Rand, H. (2006). *Narradrama: Drama therapy, narrative and the creative arts* (2nd ed.). Possibilities Press.

Fredrickson, B. L. (2009). *Positivity*. Crown Publishers.

Fredrickson, B. L. (2013). Updated thinking on positivity ratios. *American Psychologist, 68*(9), 814–822. https://doi.org/10.1037/a0033584

Fredrickson, B. L., Cohn, M. A., Coffey, K. A., Pek, J., & Finkel, S. M. (2008). Open hearts build lives: Positive emotions, induced through loving-kindness meditation, build consequential personal resources. *Journal of Personality and Social Psychology, 95*(5), 1045–1062. https://doi.org/10.1037/a0013262

Paulus, D. (2020). American repertory theatre. Cited in the *Harvard Gazette*. https://news.harvard.edu/gazette/story/2020/10/american-repertory-theater-announces-falls-virtual-programming/

Pavior, S., & Angus, L. (2017). *Narrative processes in emotion focused therapy for trauma*. APA.

Quoidbach, J., Gruber, J., Mikolajczak, M., Kogan, A., Kotsou, I., & Norton, M. I. (2014). Emodiversity and the emotional ecosystem. *Journal of Experimental Psychology, 143*(6), 2057–2066. https://doi.org/10.1037/a0038025

Ramsey, H. L., Young, K., & Tarulli, D. (2010). Scaffolding and concept formation in narrative therapy: A qualitative research report. *Journal of System Therapies, 29*(4), 74–91.

Zimmerman, J., & Beaudoin, M. M. (2015). Neurobiology for your narrative: How brain science can influence narrative work. *Journal of Systemic Therapies, 34*(2), 59–74.

4 Dramatherapy with adolescents in Malaysia

Be

Vanitha Chandrasegaram

> "Imagination is in fact, the central engine of meaning."
> (Blair, 2009)

Be is the title of a performance created by seven drama students at the International School of Kuala Lumpur (ISKL) in Malaysia. They worked together in drama classes at school. Their drama teacher thought their work might be enhanced by experiencing a series of sessions of dramatherapy. The focus of these sessions was on their personal development with the possibility this might contribute to the content or the development of the performance piece.

Malaysia is a multicultural country, with the population consisting predominantly of ethnic Malays, Chinese, and Indians. Kuala Lumpur is the capital of Malaysia, with a population of 1.808 million (2021). Malaysia has a total population of 32.37 million (2021). Kuala Lumpur, like many other capital cities around the world, hosts many local and international businesses with 10% of the population being expatriates. ISKL is part of a worldwide network. As such, it provides a consistent curriculum for the children of executives of international companies whose domicile may change every few years. This means that the student population may represent most major countries of the world. The school is also attended by children of local families who wish to access this type of education.

Many private colleges and universities in Malaysia are affiliated with international universities, from countries such as the United Kingdom, the United States, Australia, Canada, and India. Students who have gone through international schools are still able to continue with international degrees, in Malaysia or in other countries. English is the medium of education. Many of the teachers in the international schools are from countries such as the United States, the United Kingdom and Australia. ISKL follows the American school curriculum. It is the oldest and most respected international school in Malaysia.

DOI: 10.4324/9781003082897-8

Dramatherapy sessions

The group consisted of seven young women aged 14 to 18 years old. They originated from Malaysia, India, Iran, Japan, Vietnam, the United States, and Australia. Each session lasted for two-and-a-half hours and followed a developmental model commonly followed in dramatherapy (Jones, 1996), with this structure followed in each session:

1   Warm–up
2   Focusing
3   Main activity
4   Processing and feedback
5   Closure

The sessions took place in a drama studio. The studio was equipped with stage lighting, black curtains in the background, a sound system, and chairs. A corner of the room provided the teacher's office. This meant that we needed to transform the space into a dramatherapy space rather than a classroom. One of the ways we did that was to use warm–ups to make the space into a space for dramatherapy. Some of the warm–ups we used were movement exercises, games, and name games. The students were reminded about the intention of the sessions, which was to get to know themselves and each other better, to enhance relationships and help create the content of the school theatre performance. Working in their drama studio, gave the group access to beautiful props with which they creatively improvised to use for their performances of their stories, further prompting creative flow.

As dramatherapists we recreate spaces for group members to be free to express ideas, to move freely, to connect with others in the group, to connect with possibilities of the space. Always with the question–what could happen if we took this space over? For this group, the drama room became a space for them **not** to be working on a performance piece, to be free of the gaze of an outside audience or assessor, to be relaxed about performance as they moved from their individual space to add, combine and connect with others but still with the individual space to return to making the space their own, making it empty in order to fill it with themselves, to keep changing its shape under their own control. Peter Brook (1968) wrote, "I can take any empty space and call it a bare stage. A man walks across this empty space whilst someone is watching him, and this is all that is needed for an act of theatre to be engaged" (p. 11).

This is familiar territory for dramatherapy, and we call it warming up. We work with others in whatever space we are given and make it our own. So it becomes filled with ourselves, with us together, with new colour, focus, and activity. We become engaged physically, socially, emotionally, individually, neurologically, warming up our imaginations to enter states of flow Csikszentmihalyi (1996). In this group, we worked with our physical bodies to come alive as a whole – to feel connected with ourselves and thus able to connect with others. As we warmed up our bodies, we warmed up our minds and our social connections. From linking with our own sympathetic and parasympathetic nervous systems, we moved into a familiar dramatherapy warm-up called mirroring, in which we literally mirror the actions of a partner. Often this starts with following and then copying large to finer movements to focusing on facial expressions and mirroring those back to each other, changing from leader to follower in a fluid sequence. In our mirroring activities in dramatherapy, we are stimulating our mirror neurons which promotes empathy (Freeman, 2011). When one person follows another's body language, they start to feel more connected and so they may become more relaxed about working together. Mirroring also enables the participants to be more focused and present during the activity.

The mirroring activity helps the secretion of oxytocin, which is correlated with increased trust, reduced fear, and improved emotional regulation. This, in turn, allows participants to address traumatic and fearful experiences from the past. Previous autonomic defence systems are relaxed, which allows the participants to unlearn the maladaptive responses and allows new patterns of engagement and responses to be explored (Stewart et al., 2016).

Main activity

We used stories the group members created from picture cards which provided visual and imaginative stimuli for dramatic action, as well as a focus for group members to be working on ways to interact, make decisions together and become more spontaneous with each other in ideas and actions. It also allowed emotional connection to the participants' own stories without them needing to divulge personal material before they were ready to do so.

The main activity for the first session was to make fictional stories using picture cards and then act the stories out. Part of the pleasure of story making is the mental images that are created. "We experience the events in the story in a vivid manner by mentally stimulating the content of the story" (Martinez-Conde et al., 2019).

Using picture cards helps participants get into a state of interest or excitement about doing the activity. It helps participants have a sense of reference, a warm-up for their own sense of creativity. Staying in the fiction also allows participants to look at their stories more objectively. They can distance themselves enough to see a bigger picture which involves their interaction with each other. Staying in the fiction allows an element of fun to be expressed in the activity. Fun is welcomed in dramatherapy where it may not be in some other forms of psychotherapy. Fun and laughter release dopamine, which produces a sense of euphoria and acts as a motivator to continue the behaviour (Yim, 2016).

These are themes that emerged from the stories in the first session. Two brothers who were imprisoned indefinitely in a dungeon by an unfair king, worked together with their pet crow to steal the key and escape. A possible theme was 'working together to overcome difficulty'.

An independent queen blinded an advisor who proposed to her because she wanted to remain independent although she had warm feelings for him. Possibly a theme of the cost of being independent.

A happily married couple found out the wife was pregnant. When she went for a walk, an alluring hand began to caress her baby bump, at first gently and then very hard as a masked woman emerged and tried to kill the pregnant woman. The woman called for help from her husband who recognised his ex-girlfriend but could not stop her from killing his wife. Themes of jealousy and violence and betrayal.

While de-roling from the story roles, one participant acknowledged that the stories had prompted her to share some real concerns, high anxiety and stress about her current university applications. Group members were able to offer support with her anxieties.

At the end of that session, the participants shared that it felt very liberating that they were given the space to create any story, without any expectations or judgements. They said they had felt safe. According to Porges (2009), who developed the polyvagal theory, oxytocin is produced during social engagement. When we are present with another person, we are able to connect with them, empathise with them and are able to feel joy, connection, and love. We feel safe, secure, and in a happy place.

The second session began with physical warm-ups using yoga stretches to enhance the mind and body connection. Dramatherapy works with embodiment, which Forbes (2011) describes as being on a continuum, from exteroception, focusing on the external environment, to proprioception, with a growing awareness of where the body is in space, and interoception, with a growing awareness of what is happening within the body. This was followed by a focusing activity involving walking in ways specified by different leaders taking turns. The intention of the focusing activity was for the participants to be reacquainted with the space and with each other and to explore the feeling of moving in different ways. The playfulness in this activity resulted in a lot of laughter. Positive emotional arousal results in synaptic linkages or neuroplasticity to occur. "It opens our hearts and minds and allows us to discover and build new skills, new ties, new knowledge and new ways of being" (Fredrickson, 2009, pp. 21–24).

The main activity was mask making and self-exploration. We made masks from manila cards and used coloured pencils and coloured markers. The first masks were to depict how they see themselves, and the second masks were to reflect how they thought others saw them.

Processing and feedback

The masks appeared to give rise to reflections about individual identity and elicited more self-disclosure. Jennings (1990) says, "The way of the mask is rich and infinite and brings together both an art form in itself and a therapeutic journey for therapist and client alike" (p. 128). Common themes included some confusion in trying to integrate the many facets of the self which had appeared on the masks; some comments about the importance of ethnicity, culture, and religion and how important it was to be intelligent and seen to be intelligent. Overall, there was some difficulty in finding, defining, and owning characteristics and difficulty in articulating how they might be seen by others.

The third session took place on the last official day of school with the students tired and stressed, so we chose a gentle and familiar warm-up exercise to bring them into the space and to begin to connect with each other.

The focus was the past, present, and future, with a range of objects from which they could choose to help with warming up to this theme. The use of objects helps with movement from concrete to imagination to creation through projection onto the objects. As the session continued each person chose an object to which they felt drawn in a non-specific way.

These were often attached to childhood memories or episodic memories (Wilson, 2014), though one member chose concerns about the materialism of the world and how artificial intelligence would dominate. In the review and processing, the group members were able to share how they felt stressed, sad, and vulnerable. The objects seemed largely to have taken them back to a simpler past, but now the reality was more complicated with the weight of their worry and stress of attaining the high standards which they, and their families, had set for them. Some were applying for university places and worried about gaining entrance to the universities that promised the greatest futures. One participant was worried that she might be disowned if she did not fulfil her family's expectations. Already this had caused distress as she wanted to pursue a different course than what her family wanted for her.

There seemed to be a new closeness in the group as they listened to each other and shared how they each felt and dealt with stress. Some of them introduced apps they used for meditation techniques and mentioned yoga, listening to music, playing in a band, speaking to a mother as helpful. One group member suggested sharing her feelings with others and writing a journal about feelings.

Later we did a meditation exercise, to help the participants de-stress. Meditation reduces stress by improving self-regulation which enhances neuroplasticity and leads to health benefits. "It is proposed that the mechanism through which mindfulness meditation exerts its effects is a process of enhanced self-regulation, including attention control, emotion regulation and self-awareness" (Tang et al., 2015).

The young women said that this session had clarified fears they shared around not living up to family expectations and their own high expectations of themselves. One participant said that the session had helped her to clarify her decision to follow her heart. Another group member suggested that we think of being with ourselves instead of being by ourselves. She spoke about being a good friend to herself.

At the end, when I sent an imaginary treasure box around, most expressed appreciation for being in this group and having this space to share uncomfortable feelings and discussions.

In the fourth session, we tried a new physical warm-up, building on those they had done already. This brought in more playfulness and more connecting with each other.

The main activity was Moreno's Social Atom (Moreno, 1947) which involves mapping the people to whom they are closest and who have the most impact on their lives. They also may include those with whom they have conflict. The second part of this activity involves using others in the group to sculpt each person represented in the drawing of the social atom and letting each character say what they feel to the person who drew the social atom. The person can then communicate their feelings about each character in the social atom.

The intention of this activity is to give a view of the relationship dynamics group members have in their lives and to address any unexpressed emotions towards people who play a significant role in their life. It can help in addressing unresolved emotions and conflicts and sometimes has a cathartic effect on some of the participants.

For many of the participants, there was a common theme of missing a parent working in another country or absent from the family for other reasons. Other themes included closeness to particular family members, parents, or siblings and dynamics around that and other relatives who were once close but were not anymore. One of the participants revealed the difficulty of having a sibling with mental health challenges. Another of blaming herself for a relative moving away from her family. Another participant's theme was gratitude for having support from her community. Other themes included fear of intoxicated relatives, and of being bullied.

Stress begins with the hypothalamus–pituitary–adrenal (HPA) axis, a series of endocrine glands in the brain and on the kidneys, which control the body's reaction to stress. When our body detects a stressful situation, the HPA produces the hormone cortisol which helps us take instant action. But when the stress is continuous the activity level, the neural network, and number of neural connections is increased in the amygdala, the brain's fear center. As levels of cortisol rise, the electric signals in the hippocampus, which is the part of the brain associated with learning, memory, and stress control, deteriorates. Too much cortisol can cause the brain to shrink in size and loss of synaptic connections between neurons and the shrinking of the prefrontal cortex, the part of the brain that controls decision-making, judgement, concentration, and social interaction. It leads to fewer brain cells being made in the hippocampus, which means chronic stress might make it difficult for us to learn and remember things (Wilson, 2014).

Meditation and movement help to reverse these effects. However, while our body produces cortisol, our pituitary glands help to produce oxytocin, which is the hormone that helps us to seek support when we are stressed. Oxytocin also helps us empathise with others when they are going through a stressful period.

At the end of this section, group members suggested sitting in the circle for a few moments longer rather than rushing off to the next engagement. This indicated a degree of relaxation and comfort with each other. They respected what they had processed in this session, how it brought them closer together and made them feel more grounded with each other.

The performance

The performance became about female empowerment. This started with depictions from the 1950s of the ideal characteristics of a beautiful woman. This was all about appearance and about how women are depicted on the screen. The actors in this play showed how frustrating these stereotyped and shallow roles are, but they may be all that is offered as roles for actors who need to get work. The next scene showed women's need to fight for their rights.

Then a fairy godmother appeared to do magic with periods and the pains and moods experienced by girls/women going through the menstrual cycle. The actors turned this into a comedy with a very serious point, which they managed to make hilarious, engaging the audience through laughter while throwing sanitary products into the audience.

The final scene was from a true story of a woman who had been abused for years. The final straw was when her husband burnt her face with a hot iron. She reacted by burning her husband's feet so badly that he later died. She was sent to prison, where she continued to work to empower women.

Evaluation

Having witnessed the performance and in speaking with the students afterwards, it was clear that the dramatherapy sessions had a big impact on the development of the performance.

While no specific measures were used to identify results or outcomes from being in this dramatherapy group, effects and outcomes became clear in the group-processing time as well as in the final performance.

The group sessions were all attended by all the young women. All participated in the physical warm-up parts of the sessions. At different stages they began to become more fully part of the group, contributing ideas and actions, and becoming more willing and able to share personal material from their lives, including their emotional lives.

Each session ended with a choice of comments from an imaginary treasure chest, with the participants then having time to reflect and draw or write in their journals. They could share what they chose from the session. There was warmth and engagement as they shared coping strategies and offered the wisdom of being one's own best friend. There seemed to be relief in discovering that they were each dealing with major life changes and decisions and that they felt the weight of family expectations in choosing a life path. Some commented that it had been wonderful to be able to have a free hand in creating and enacting, without having to follow a set script, and how liberating to have no expectations or judgements about their stories, their acting, or what they shared in the group. This indicated that participation in the dramatherapy group had offered a different experience to that offered by the drama class. The students had reported to the drama teacher that they felt much closer to each other after the dramatherapy sessions and that this made it easier to work creatively together. The dramatherapist commented on the maturity and combined wisdom of the young women in the way they were able to share emotions, space, and ideas generously with each other. The drama teacher reported positively on the performance, from the profundity of the themes and the skilful and lighthearted way they had dealt with serious themes.

They had written the script for their performance themselves and did all their preparation within two weeks. This was the shortest time ever for them to have developed a performance. This indicated that there had been synergy and flow within this group, which they had not always experienced.

Generally, the message from each of them was how they became connected to themselves as well as each other. They reported that the sessions had created a safe space for them to just be, hence the title of the performance: *Be*.

Conclusion

These sessions of dramatherapy were arranged to gauge the response of a group of young women aged 14 to 19 to a series of six dramatherapy sessions. The intention was to help the student actors access their deeper selves in order to create a theatre performance which was meaningful to them and resonated with what they had experienced or might be experiencing in their lives. Participation in the dramatherapy group was found to have a significant impact on the school project. The result was a powerful performance, where none of the content of the sessions was represented directly in the play but where the new content of the play arose out of the close relationships and freedom of expression the dramatherapy sessions had allowed.

Acknowledgements

I would like to thank Mr. Timothy Howe, drama teacher, for giving me the opportunity to work with his drama students.

I would also like to thank the International School of Kuala Lumpur for being open to having dramatherapy personal development sessions with their students.

References

Blair, R. (2009). Cognitive neuroscience and acting: Imagination, conceptual blending, and empathy. *The drama review, 53*(4), 93–103.
Brook, P. (1968). *The empty space*. Pelican.
Csikszentmihalyi, M. (1996). *Creativity: Flow and the psychology of discovery and invention*. Harper Collins.

Department of Statistics Malaysia Official Portal. (2021). https://www.dosm.gov.my/v1/index.php?r=column/cthemeByCat&cat=155&bul_id=OVByWjg5YkQ3MWFZRTN5bDJiaEVhZz09&menu_id=L0pheU43NWJwRWVSZklWdzQ4TlhUUT09

Forbes, B. (2011). Interoception: Mindfulness in the body: The continuum of embodiment. *LAYoga*, May, 56.

Fredrickson, B. L. (2009). *Positivity*. Crown Publishing Group.

Freeman, B. (2011). The social neuroscience of empathy in the theatre of global ethics. *Performing Ethos: International Journal of Ethics in Theatre & Performance*, *2*(1), 41–54. https://doi.org/10.1386/peet.2.1.41_1

Jennings, S. (1990). *Dramatherapy with families, groups and individuals: Waiting in the wings*. Jessica Kingsley.

Jones, P. (1996). *Drama as therapy: Theatre as living*. Psychology Press.

Martinez-Conde, S., Alexander, R. G., Blum, D., Britton, N., Lipska, B. K., Quirk, G. J., & Macknik, S. L. (2019). The storytelling brain: How neuroscience stories help bridge the gap between research and society. *Journal of Neuroscience*, *39*(42), 8285–8290. https://doi.org/10.1523/JNEUROSCI.1180-19.2019

Moreno, J. L. (1947). Organization of the social atom. *Sociometry*, *10*(3), 287–293. https://doi.org/10.2307/2785079

Porges, S. W. (2009). Stress and parasympathetic control. *Stress Science: Neuroendocrinology*, 306–312.

Stewart, A. L., Field, T. A., & Echterling, L. G. (2016). Neuroscience and the magic of play therapy. *International Journal of Play Therapy*, *25*(1), 4. https://doi.org/10.1037/pla0000016

Tang, Y. Y., Holzel, B. K., & Posner, M. I. (2015). The neuroscience of mindfulness meditation. *Nature Reviews Neuroscience*, 1–13. doi:10.1038/nrn3916

Wilson, R. Z. (2014). *Neuroscience for counsellors: Practical applications for counsellors, therapists and mental health practitioners*. Jessica Kingsley.

Yim, J. E. (2016). Therapeutic benefits of laughter in mental health: A theoretical review. *Tohoku Journal of Experimental Medicine*, *239*(3), 244–249. https://pubmed.ncbi.nlm.nih.gov/27439375

5 A multi-theoretical, multimodal arts-psychotherapy approach to trauma and depression

Agnès Desombiaux-Sigley

Introduction

The philosophy that underpins and supports my integrative arts psycho-therapy approach is grounded in Merleau-Ponty's (1962; Abram, 1997) phenomenology of perception, which prioritises the experience of the 'lived body' as the primary instrument to understand others. Psychody-namic (McWilliams, 2020; Schore, 2001, 2019) and attachment theories (Cozolino, 2002, 2012; Karen, 1998) inform the development of the thera-peutic relationship at the centre of the therapeutic process. The meth-ods woven through the process and their underpinning theories are based on mindfulness meditation practice and visualisation (Kabat Zinn, 2005a, 2005b; Williams et al., 2007) as tools for self-awareness, self-regulation, and self-compassion and psychosomatic integration (PSI) for complex trauma and dissociation (Lightstone & Suebert, 2009), a form of sensorimotor psy-chotherapy (Ogden et al., 2006) that draws from somatic therapies (Kurtz, 1990; Levine, 2008), neurosciences (Perry & Szalavitz, 2006; Porges, 2011; Schore, 2019; Siegel, 2006, 2020), trauma theory (Herman, 1992; Roths-child, 2000; Briere & Scott, 2012; Van der Kolk, 2014;), and ego states theory (Watkins & Watkins, 1997), which acknowledges that a person has different parts of the self that take on different roles and functions (some-times conflictual) and that these parts have different developmental needs (Schmidt, 2009).

The arts-psychotherapy process (McNiff, 1992; Robbins, 2000; Pearson & Wilson, 2009), mostly non-directive in the case study presented, provides a choice of materials consisting of a sand tray and an extensive collection of sym-bols (Jung, 1997; Amman, 1991; Kalf, 2003; Pattis Zoja, 2004; Weinrib, 2004; Turner, 2005); a range of drawing pastels, crayons, paint, and collage material, paper, plasticine, and clay (Malchiodi, 2002, 2006); and dance and movement therapy (Halprin, 2005). Some of this work is underpinned by Gestalt (Perls, 1992) and dreamwork (Freud, 1955, 2010; Jung, 2003).

DOI: 10.4324/9781003082897-9

Case study

Dynamic formulation

Madeleine presented with symptoms of depression, anxiety, and post-traumatic stress disorder, which were consistent with her early life history. She had early experiences of disrupted attachment through her mother's grief, neglect, and abandonment and then physical and emotional abuse from her mother as an unpredictable alcoholic. These early experiences failed to give her an internal basic sense of safety and security and contributed to her fragmented sense of self, lack of boundaries, dissociation, anxiety, and lack of a sense of purpose (McWilliams, 2020). As a toddler she may have experienced a sense of inadequacy, shame, and self-doubt, as described by Erikson and Erikson (1998); these feelings were still with her in her adult life. Many researchers agree on the effect of trauma on the developing brain (Cozolino, 2012; Siegel, 2020; Schore, 1994, 2001). Perry and Szalavitz (2006) explain:

> The most traumatic aspects of all disasters involve the shattering of human connections. And this is especially true for children. Being harmed by the people who are supposed to love you, being abandoned by them, being robbed by the one-on-one relationship that allows you to feel safe and valued and to become humane – these are profoundly destructive experiences.
>
> (p. 231)

Madeleine's depression symptoms stemmed from cultural bereavement and transgenerational grief, expressed through an overwhelming and pervasive feeling of sadness, with flat affect and prosody. Protective factors were other maternal figures, a grandmother and an aunt; her love for learning, creativity, and art; and her intelligence. Madeleine had a symbiotic relationship with her younger sister which created a tendency to develop co-dependency in adult life. The attachment trauma (anxious/avoidant) was originally relational, and so the relationship with the therapist, with whom she could express her childhood trauma in her first language and with whom she shared the same culture, had potential as an important role in the healing process (Carlson, 1979; Griner & Smith, 2006). Over three-and-a-half-years, Madeleine came to therapy sessions weekly for two years and then fortnightly, for a total of 75 sessions. The images and artwork presented in this chapter, those most significant or indicative of her process (Miller, 2014), helped her express her internal experiences at the time and construct a narrative of her past experiences to make sense of different stages of her life still at play in her unconscious and in her body. The integrative arts psychotherapy process facilitated the emergence of unconscious material as stated in McNiff (1992): "The process of talking with images is close to the free association techniques of early psychoanalysis, which enable unconscious expressions to circumvent the conscious mind" (p. 106).

The images in the space between us connected us, and I had an intense physical response (somatic countertransference) to each of them that gave me a powerful indication of her internal state. Artmaking often happened in silence; we communicated through her artwork, with symbolism and metaphors, using both the conscious left brain and the unconscious right brain (Schore, 2019). Research in trauma and neurobiology shows increasingly that it is through the exchange between the emotions felt through the body of the patient and the therapist that deep healing occurs (Rothschild, 2017; Pert, 1997; Herman, 1992 [2015]; Van der Kolk, 2014).

My role was to attend and provide a sense of sufficient safety (Herman, 1992 [2015]; Rothschild, 2017) for her to bring her vulnerable parts (including child parts) and painful memories in her own time and within the structure of regular sessions. My main focus was to attune to the expression of her emotions and promote social engagement through our subtle body interactions: body language, facial expressions, gaze, and tone of voice (Porges, 2011). A nurturing aspect of her mother was her artistic expression; a painter herself, she had encouraged creativity in her children. The creative process can have the role of a transitional object (Winnicott, 2006). Her mother tongue and creativity were like an oxygen mask. She stated that in our sessions, she found the breath of life.

Leaving the theoretical framework in the background, I entered each session with a grounded mindful awareness of the present moment, tuning with all my senses into her experience of being in the world through the somatic, motoric, imaginal, visual, and verbal expression of our intersubjective relationship (Lecours & Bouchard, 1997, as cited in Quatman, 2015, p. 34).

As I worked with Madeleine, I experienced intense body responses on many occasions. For this chapter, I have decided to focus on my own somatic responses to her artwork, in a reflexive process, alongside the verbal session notes.

Early stages: a sense of self

With the first image she produced, I had a resonance through my body: deep pain, an ache in my core, torment, agitation, and deep sadness. I shed tears with her when she expressed the terror she felt with her sister during a violent incident involving her mother. I made space for compassion through the opening of my heart, and a desire to envelop her with the gentleness she needed at the time. These intense feelings and sensations foster the early stage and formation of the therapeutic alliance through conscious and unconscious processes. Schore (2007) emphasises that recent research in developmental science and neuroscience have demonstrated the role of the relational-emotional contact between humans and the impact of this process on the part of the brain that regulates bodily based survival functions. Schore (2007) noted that

> [t]he current paradigm shift into the nonconscious affective relational functions of the right brain has direct bearing upon the underlying of the change process as it is expressed in the intersubjective field. This

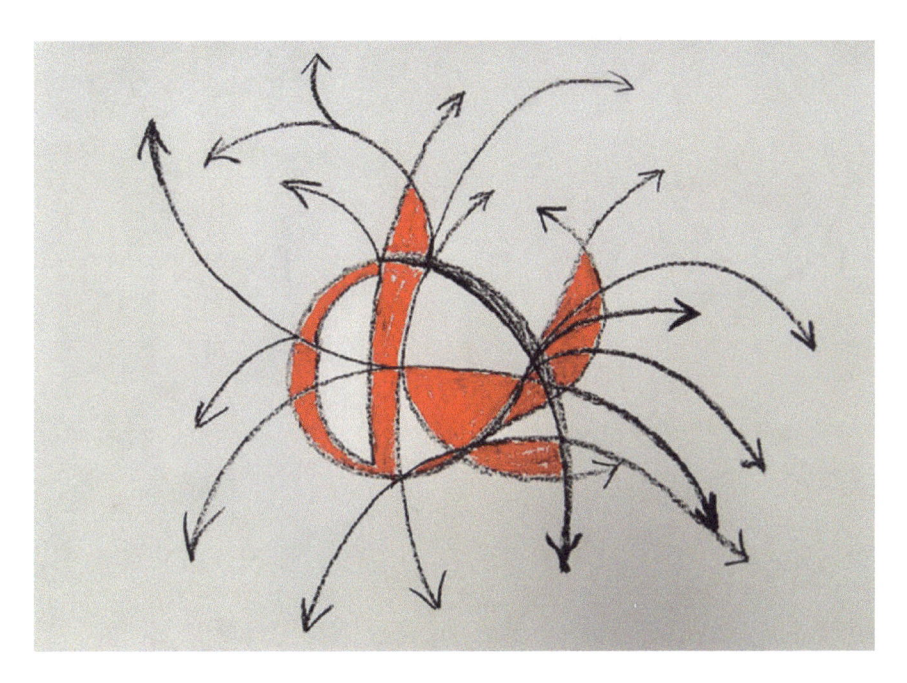

Figure 5.1 A sense of self (oil pastels, session 1)

perspective highlights the clinician's role as a co-participant in the creation of the therapeutic alliance, and as regulator of the patient's dysregulated affective states.

(p. 7)

Transgenerational grief

Madeleine: *"The hangman is me, I used to draw hangmen all the time as a teenager".* She said that her maternal grandfather committed suicide (by hanging) and her mother lost a baby (at eight months) when Madeleine was still a toddler; the mother was grieving before and after Madeleine's own birth. Black birds flowing from a womb, the orange sun, creativity, potential, green pasture, and hope; there is life and joy in the environment, as well as softness. There was already sadness when she was in the womb. New life and death are intertwined.

Her sadness enveloped me. I felt a heavy weight on my heart: it is the sadness and grief carried by three generations of women in her family. Attuned to her emotions, her story of grief and loss resonated with aspects of my own.

Stern (2004) explains that our nervous system is constructed to be captured by the nervous system of others so that we can experience others as if from

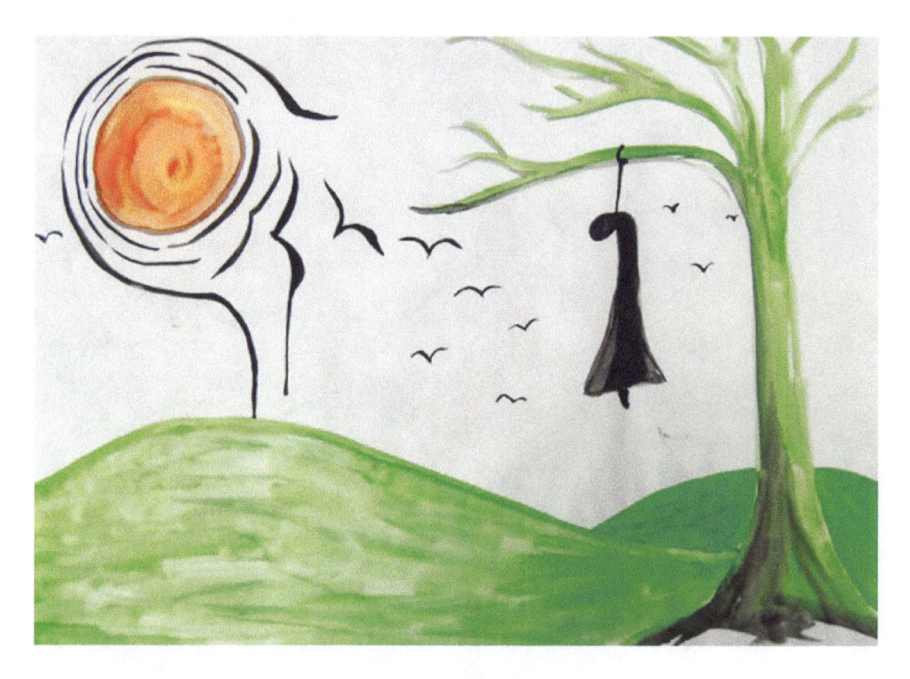

Figure 5.2 A hanged man (watercolour, session 3)

within their skin, as well as from within our own. A direct feeling route into the other person is potentially open, and we resonate with and participate in their experience, and they in ours. We are able to read other people's intentions and feelings within our bodies.

I encouraged Madeleine all through the therapeutic process to connect with her body sensations and her felt sense (Gendlin, 1998; Kurtz, 1990; Levine, 2008; Mehling et al., 2011). Siegel (2020) and Liebermann et al. (2007) have indicated that the process of putting feelings and sensations into words affects labelling, helps manage negative emotional experience, enables the left and right brain to become more integrated, and helps with the regulation of emotional arousal. Schore (2012, pp. 7–8) states that

> [w]ith respect to the paradigm shift towards relationally oriented psychotherapy, clinical interpersonal neurobiological models of therapeutic change are now moving from left brain to right brain, from the mind to the body, and from the central to the autonomic nervous system. This shift in paradigm into relational models of psychotherapy is being paralleled in social neuroscience studies of the essential role of the right brain in social interaction. Indeed, there is now a call to 'move from the classical one-brain neuroscience toward a novel two-body approach'.
>
> (Dumas, 2011, p. 349)

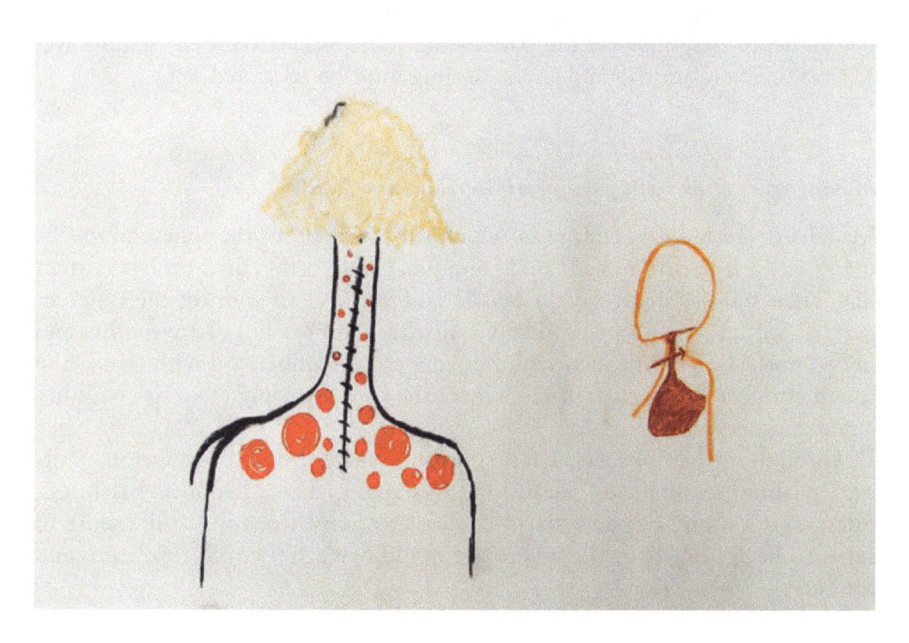

Figure 5.3 My mother and me (oil pastel, session 4)

The main attachment figure

Madeleine: *"This is my mother and me. The only time we were allowed to touch her was when we were in the car; she would request a massage from us. She was very tight and bony. I remember loving these rare moments of tenderness where I could touch her. . . . I felt my mother's pain and vulnerability and would feel compassion for her and at the same time she was inaccessible: she could not see me, and I could not see her. . . . I was on the back seat. This is me on the right-hand side."*

Madeleine could not develop, breathe, talk, or be heard or seen for who she was. She was deprived of the gaze of her mother; therefore, she had no eyes. She was deprived of caring communication with her mother; therefore, she had no mouth or ears. As her voice softened and lowered, I felt a void, pain, disconnection, and numbness – a little child who needed rocking, cuddling, and a soft voice. I sensed that my whole being was adapting to a child's need and our voices and bodies were in tune. The creative process became her transitional object (Winnicott, 2006) and would be for the duration of the therapy, as a soothing object connected to the mother, the mother tongue, and the motherland. There was hope we might achieve attachment repair as described by Schore (2019):

> In my model of 'relational trauma' I have suggested that it is not just misattunements that lead to the traumatic predisposition. It is also the lack of

repair, and that repair and interactive regulation requires a very personal, authentic response on the part of the therapist. Attachment trauma was originally relational, and so the healing must be relational.

(p. 268)

Making sense of the split parts of self in relation to family

Madeleine created this collage in which she worked out the different attachments to each person in the family and what impact they had on her current life. Then she decided to use a needle and a thread to connect the different parts of self on the collage. While working through the links between her and her parents, she got in touch with her craving for connection with them. She found comfort in her current life, where she was nurturing close ties with her aunty and her sister.

Throughout her process, I felt splitting, cutting, death, starvation, pulling, pushing, hesitation, confusion, loss, pain, disconnection, harshness, quest, and longing but also warmth, fun, creativity, freedom, and a sense of relief to have found a space where she could bring her confusion, pain, and longing.

Hass-Cohen and Carr (2008) explain that one of the experiences of trauma in the body is a feeling of helplessness and being cut off from the language. The early stage of the therapeutic alliance and the arts process, grounded in

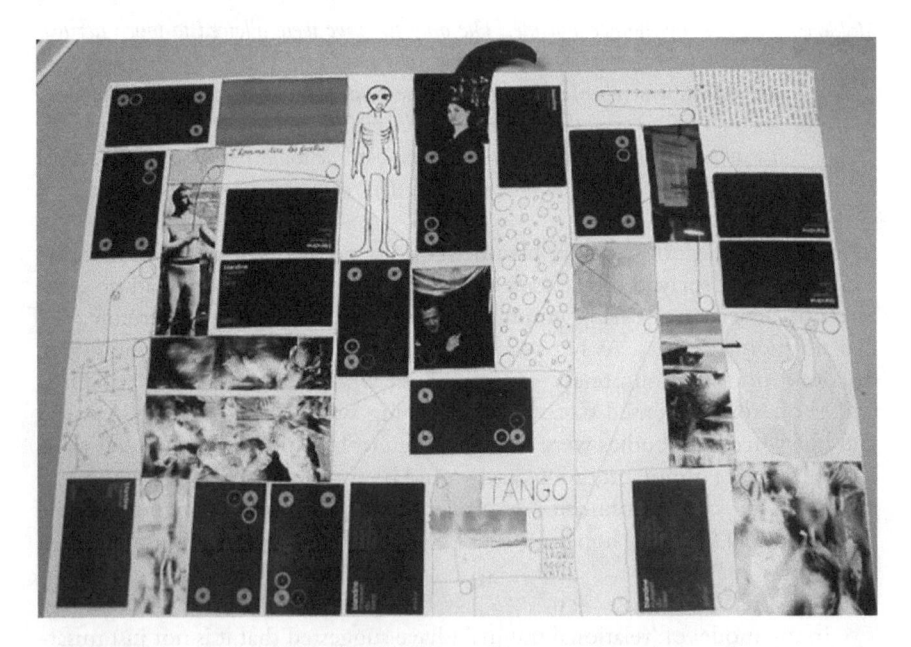

Figure 5.4 Attachment (collage, gel pen, felt, ribbon, sessions 13/14/15/16)

affective-sensory experiences, provided relief through the expression of emotions and the kinaesthetic actions required for the artwork completion.

The early affective relationship between the primary caregiver and the infant shapes the infant's emotional brain by defining the neural network connectivity and preparing them/him/her for development and maturation (Perry & Szalavitz, 2006). Working through attachment within the careful observation of the transference gave me an insight into the different attachments she might have experienced: disorganised and anxious with her mother, preoccupied with the father, symbiotic with the sister, secure with the grandmother. These different attachments repeated in her current life with people of significance (Karen, 1998) and were enacted in the transference (and countertransference) at different stages of the process.

Writing for healing cultural bereavement (paper and pen, wooden box, session 18)

Living in New Zealand, and having to express herself in a foreign language, was increasing Madeleine's sense of loss. Her mother tongue, her native language, had been central to the development of her identity, inner strength, and sense of belonging. We discussed ways for her to make space for creative writing in her busy life.

I sensed her relief, joy, and gratitude, with increased acceptance and strengthening of her sense of self. I resonated with her experience as creative writing had been a life-saving resource in my first years as a migrant. Our interpersonal connection was palpable. As Siegel (2012 [2020]) explains, the human brain has evolved with a system that is vital in interpersonal connection. Certain neurons have 'mirror' properties that link the perception of others to one's own internal state simulation. These mirror neurons shape our own actions and feelings so that we feel inside our bodies a state similar to that of the other person. "In essence, we come to resonate with the other person and the two 'me's' becomes 'we'" (Siegel (2012 [2020], p. 308).

Hass Cohen and Findlay (2015) state that "[t]he crescendo of interpersonal mirroring leads to knowing the other and, under the right social conditions, contributes to acceptance: I know and accept you" (p. 364). They explain that shared cultural understanding, intersubjective resonance, and interpersonal connectivity will favour empathy and compassion in the therapist, and resilience in the patient.

Theme of death and rebirth (sessions 23/24/25)

After a short break, Madeleine returned from France with the realisation that Aotearoa New Zealand was a necessary distant sanctuary for her healing process. In the following session, she related a powerful dream on the theme of death and rebirth that we discussed (Freud, 1955, 2010). In session 25, she acknowledged that the new sense of stability and security was bringing some

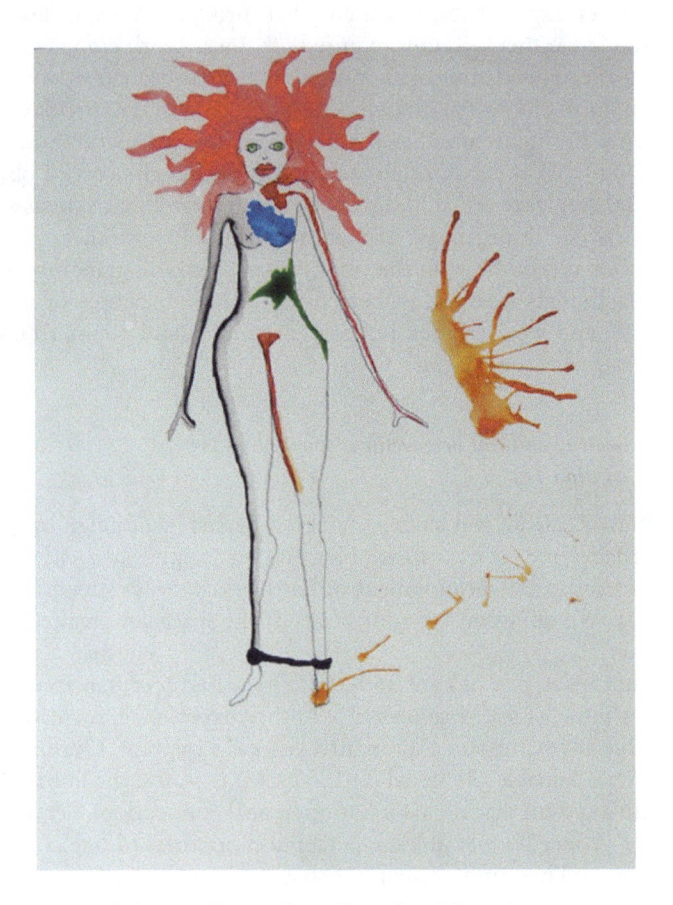

Figure 5.5 Panic attack (watercolour and pencil, session 26)

anxiety, as she was worried chaos would come back and maybe that was prefer-
able as it was known territory.

On Good Friday, Madeleine's husband announced that he was going away
for work for two weeks. She felt very anxious about staying alone with the
children and experienced a panic attack. In her subsequent drawing, an electric charge was running through her body, and she could feel her blood flow.
Madeleine felt alive (as opposed to numb/dissociated). She said she recovered
her sense of touch, realising that it had been missing. There was sadness in her
heart (blue) and something green, a sick feeling in her liver. Her feet were tied
up, she felt trapped and had let go of something dead in her.

I sensed an awakening (from the freeze response to trauma), a jolt, a wakeup
call, a life-giving current, and anger. I was touched by her reconnection to her
natural beauty, femininity, vulnerability, and naked truthfulness. Her anxiety
was palpable.

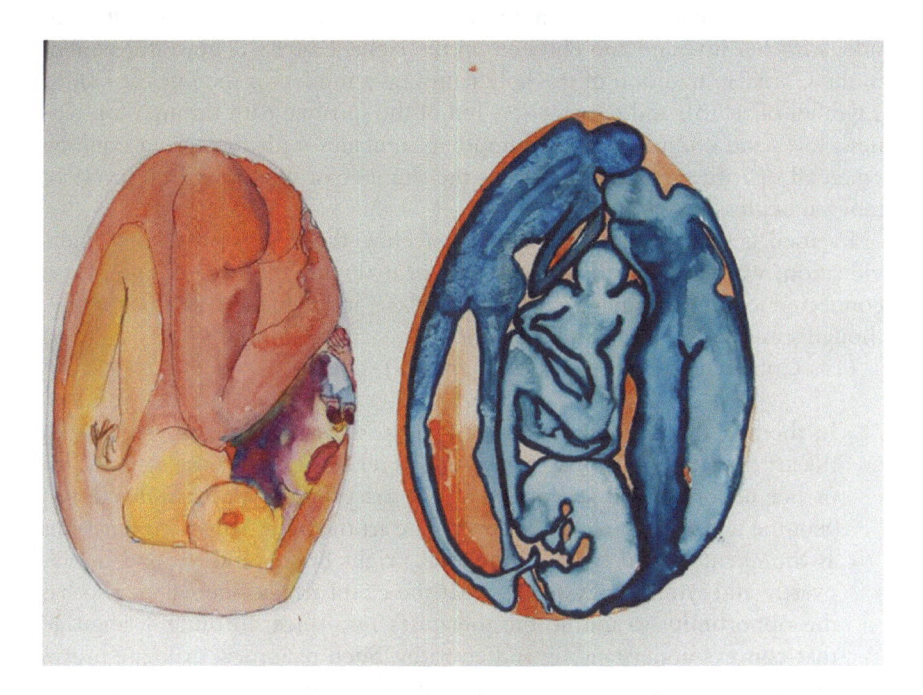

Figure 5.6 Easter (watercolour, sessions 27/28/29)

The fear of abandonment in the absence of her partner was reactivating her trauma through her sympathetic nervous system response. Porges, who developed the polyvagal theory (2011), explains that people in a dissociated state have activated the dorsal vagal complex in the brainstem, bringing about a slowdown, numbing state. He demonstrates that if therapists focus on deepening the social engagement (increase eye contact, soften gaze and prosody), it will activate the frontal vagus nerve, the major nerve of the parasympathetic nervous system (PNS) and provide an increased sense of safety in relationships. They are two major branches of the PNS, and the most recent in our evolution (myelinated) is the one linked to the cranial nerves that control facial expression and vocalisation and regulates heart and lung function.

Madeleine was deprived of touch as a child and therefore became partly numb and disconnected from her body. Siegel (2020) explains that touch is an extremely important part of the parent–child relationship, as it shapes electrical brain activity (p. 308). Gerhardt (2004, p. 205) states that a sense of safety and acceptance is provided by touch in early infancy. For Madeleine, recovering her sense of touch was a sign that she was making another step towards her sense of safety in the world, acceptance of herself, and recovery from trauma.

The three paintings (Figures 5.5, 5.6, and 5.7) were created around Easter and her birthday, as Madeleine was voicing more freely her desires and needs, which had an impact on the family dynamic. Madeleine was on the left-hand side, with her husband and children on the right. Easter is a powerful symbol in the Christian tradition of the holy family, as a model for the nuclear family, a symbol of rebirth and resurrection and of the spiritual path through forgiveness, love, and compassion. In Europe, it coincides with the spring equinox when all of nature is awakened from the slumber of winter and the cycle of renewal begins.

I sensed gestation, tightness, holding, feeling the edge of the body, individuation, warmth, rebirth, and the pain of it (Figure 5.6); regrouping, close connectedness, containment; creating her place, individuation, and belonging, though some shared (blue bodies) sadness.

Hass Cohen (as cited in King, 2016, p. 127) states,

> In therapy, the development of self-compassion and empathy starts with the art therapist's sensitivity to embedded relational media transactions, his or her unconditional acceptance of the art product, and transmission of genuine interest, caring, and respect. The art therapist, who then functions as the client's 'third hand', 'third eye', 'right brain', and 'second mind', overtly and symbolically senses what the client needs. The client also has the opportunity to mimic the therapist's resonance, forming a language that conveys understanding and empathy. Such reciprocal dialogue moves the client towards felt and anticipated aid. In art therapy, neurobiological activation in response to implied and actual movement, in particular mirror neuron and mirroring systems, evoke empathising, compassion, pleasure, and joy. These mirroring responses embody empathic reaction to art. Other involved systems include the integration of right and left hemispheric functions, bottom-up arousal and top-down regulation, and balanced activation of positive reward system activation.

An embodied/incarnated sense of self

This painting came in a reflective session about past events where Madeleine had to face her deepest fears.

My somatic reaction to this painting was joy, the picture felt alive (earth, clay, and skin): a naked body, truthful, vulnerable, confused, uncertain, surprised, and trustful, open to possibilities but hesitant to take its first steps. I felt amazed at the transformational process. The skeleton in the collage now had flesh, the beginning of an incarnation and an embodiment of her sense of self. Helping Madeleine to focus on her body sensations, as she spoke about her experiences, and the practice of mindful breathing increased her ability for self-awareness.

This process is particularly powerful for survivors of trauma as it helps improve mastery over non-verbal communications, automatic reactions, and grounding and coping skills needed to regulate frequent experiences of both

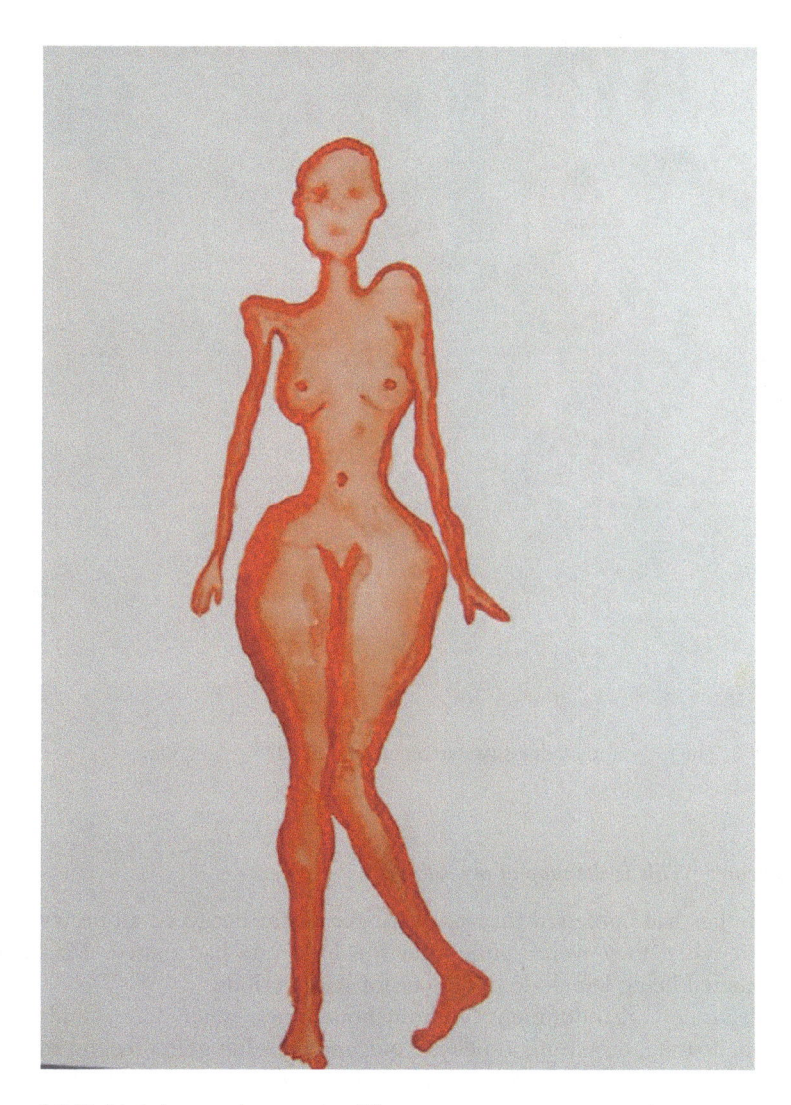

Figure 5.7 Rebirth (watercolour, session 30)

hyper-activation (overwhelm) and hypo-activation (dissociation). Ogden et al. (2006) explain that using a sensory motor psychotherapy model actively incorporates awareness of the body into clinical practice, targeting the habits of physical action, autonomic dysregulation, and posture. By addressing the physical, as well as the psychological effects of adverse experience on mind and body, sensory motor processing supports a deep, effective, and unified approach to healing.

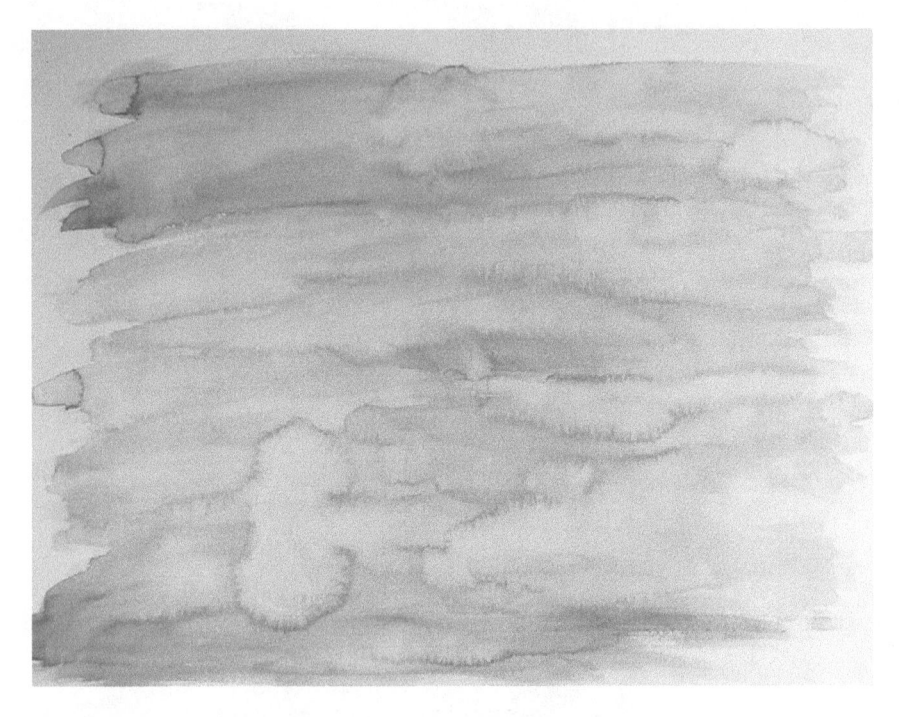

Figure 5.8 The map of my sadness (watercolour, session 32)

Madeleine: "This is the map of my sadness"

Her mother had confessed that it felt dangerous for her to be alone with her children when they were young after the little one had passed. Madeleine remembered being left alone in her cot for long periods.

I felt sadness, abandonment, without boundaries, water, tears, fluidity, no holding, floating, drowning, timeless, void, and the adult in her feeling angry: a pre-verbal memory of abandonment, surrounded by grief; a small body, a baby, or a toddler in her cot waiting for an absent mother who could neither hold her nor nurture her and who left her to cry far too long. Madeleine was in the process of individuation, and at the same time, she had this body memory (an embodied self-awareness of herself as a baby) of what had hindered some of the essential development of her sense of self.

Gerhardt (2004) demonstrates how early experience can alter brain chemistry. Lacking an early experience of blissful, protected infancy does not just affect the stress response and the ability to switch off cortisol; it can have other negative biochemical effects on the brain, such as a lack of capacity for emotional regulation. This lack often leads to adult depression, and the core of depression is a fragile sense of self.

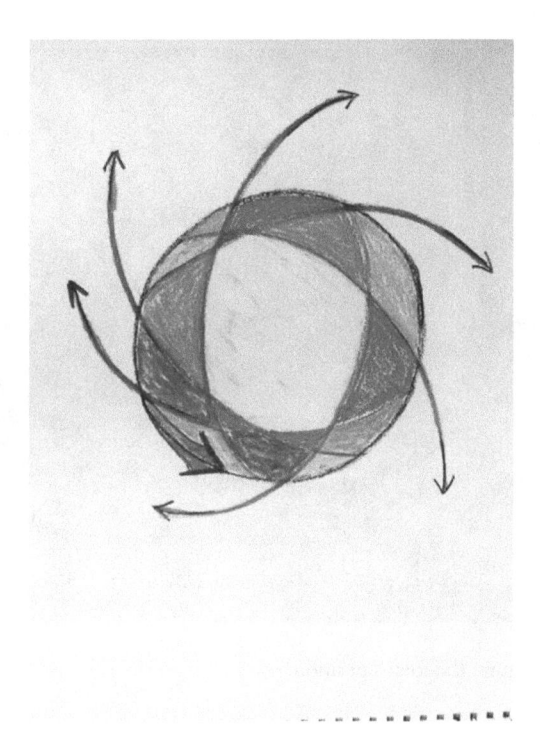

Figure 5.9 A more integrated sense of self (oil pastel, session 34)

Madeleine acknowledged she felt a more solid inner sense of stability and security and was embracing it.

My somatic response felt grounded, solid, purposeful, together, whole, joyful, a sense of ease and relief, more integrated, hopeful. I felt a beginning of motion, concentrated energy, and direction. It was starting to be clear that the creative therapeutic process had played an important role, as Winnicott (2006) wrote: "It is in playing and only in playing that the individual child or adult is able to be creative and to use the whole personality, and it is only in being creative that the individual discovers the self" (pp. 72–73).

Consolidation

About the foetus position (Figure 5.10), Madeleine said: "*I feel I am regressing, not standing on my two feet*". About the apple core (Figure 5.11), she reflected: "*There is something solid in that core*". The next clay figure was a kind of crown (Figure 5.12) with a core inside: "*With not much substance*", she reflected. "*It has lots of arms but it is not achieving anything, it is incapacitated. . . . It has a tail . . . it reminds me of my mother's alcoholism. I read somewhere that alcoholics dream of rats. The tail is her; she is still attached to me*".

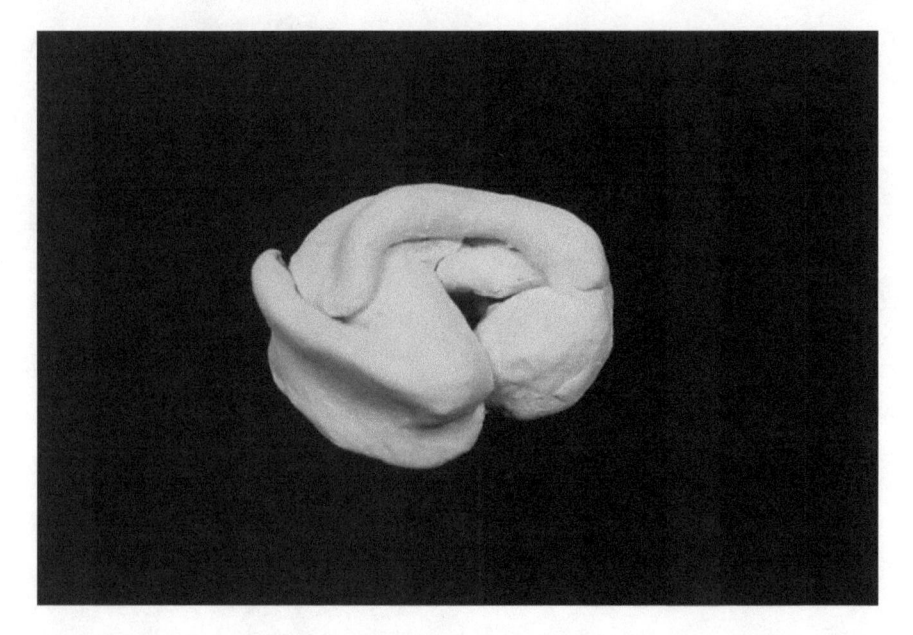

Figure 5.10 Clay figure: the foetus position

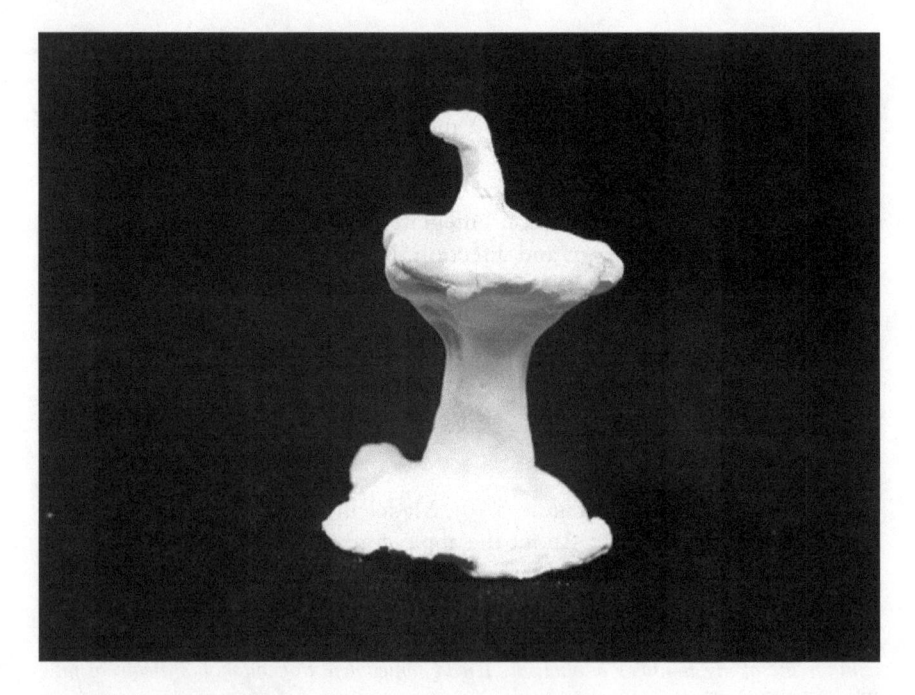

Figure 5.11 Clay figure: the core

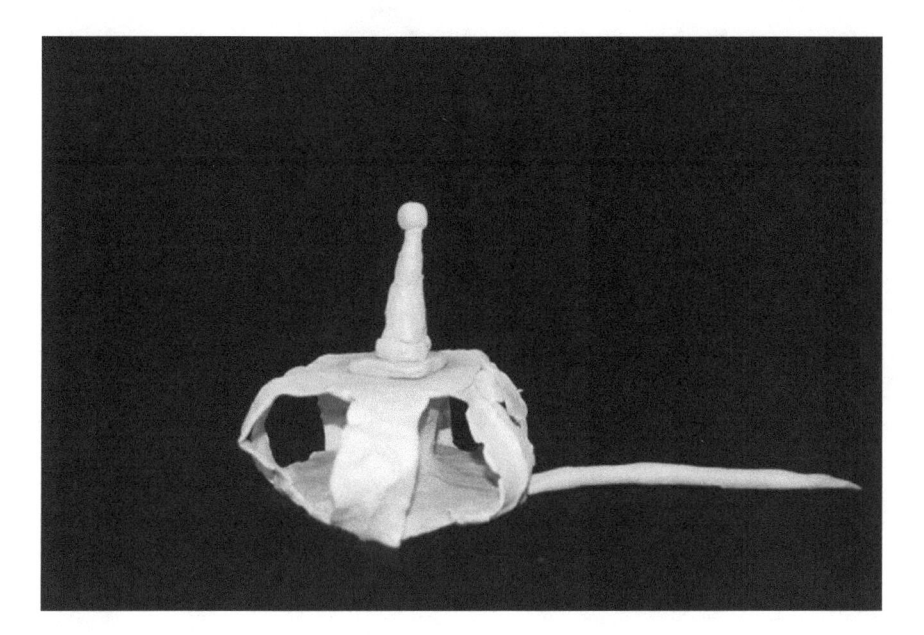

Figure 5.12 Clay figure: the crown

My experience of these artworks was to feel a sense of consolidation, solidity, tightening, hardening, holding on, holding it together, solid core self, realness, and stillness but with some residual shame and emptiness. Madeleine was getting in touch with her sense of inertia. At the same time, there was the crown from the early collage, a recurrent theme for potential. I felt I had (symbolically) to hold her hand and help her take her first steps in the world.

Robbins (1994) explains that clay is a powerful medium for engaging the client physically by stimulating the primary sensory experience (especially smell and touch). It aids in the regression to an early stage, of a budding ego when symbolisation develops.

To encourage left brain and right brain integration and strengthening of the ego, I suggested a more directed exercise that focused on resourcing the client (Figure 5.13) by bringing to the forefront internal strengths, such as the protective, the nurturing and the spiritual or core self, and connecting them to body sensations and feelings. This structured process attempted to create coherence among multiple selves across times and context, to invite connection with different parts of self and linking past and present embodied experiences (sensations and emotions) and mind through narratives (Schmidt, 2009).

Sadness, for the first time, was outside (blue circle). As it was hard for her to bring up a feeling of nurturance, I encouraged Madeleine to bring her knitting to sessions to reconnect with the sensation of caring, loving

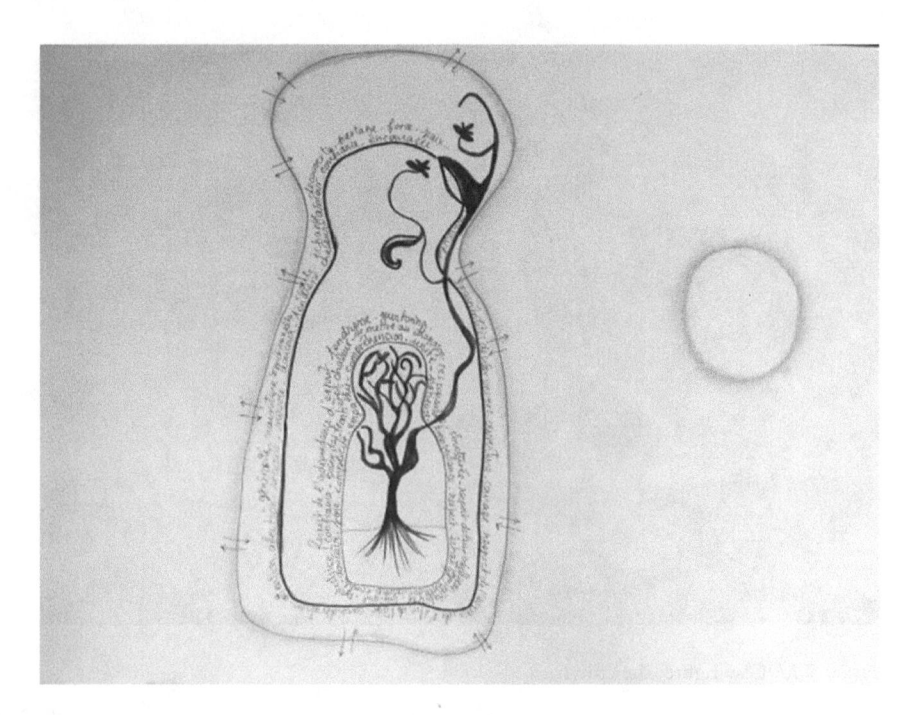

Figure 5.13 Resourcing (gel pen, sessions 46/47/48)

attention from her grandmother; softness and gentleness came alive in the room between us and in us. The sensations felt while knitting brought other memories such as the symbiotic bond she had forged with her younger sister.

She remembered a story her maternal grandmother had told her: "*She lost a lot of family members because of the war and was separated from the rest of her family when she immigrated to France after the war. She also lost a baby. I realised that I am afraid of dying away from my sister*". Madeleine has been able to make sense of her own grief and sadness through understanding the grief of all the maternal figures in her life (Kempson et al., 2008).

In Session 56, Madeleine said, "*For the first time in my life I feel like an adult. My sense of smell has come back*". Madeleine had welcomed into her home a young cousin (a teenager), an encounter which had facilitated the connection with her own inner teenager.

Siegel (2020) stated: "Self-organisation at the level of the mind must involve the integrative processing of multiple self-states across time and context. It is at the moments of transition that new self-organisational forms can be constructed" (2020, p. 356).

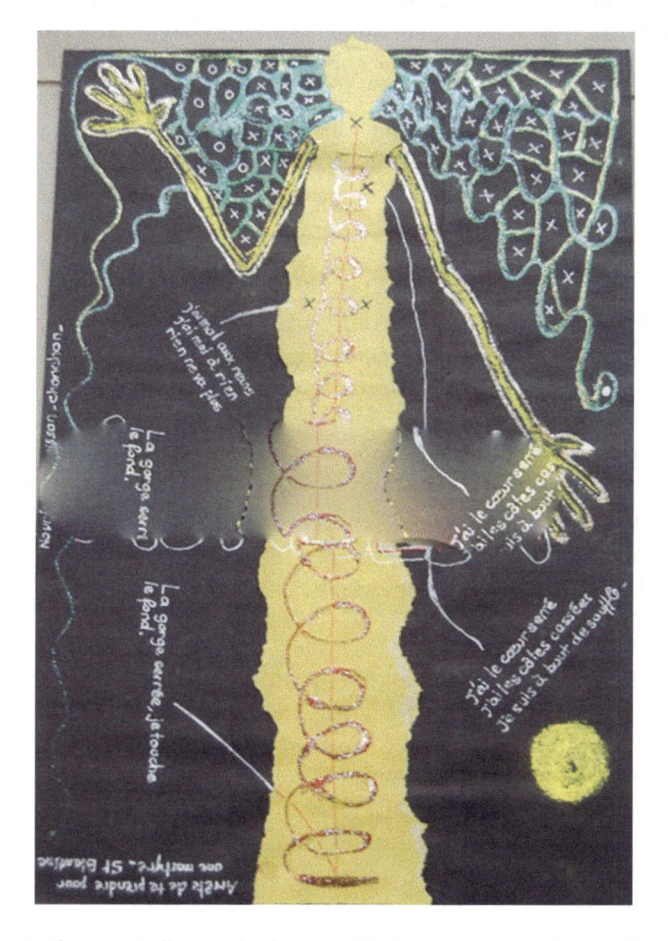

Figure 5.14 Little sister (collage and gel pen on black paper, sessions 60, 61, 62)

The internalised sick and frozen body

Madeleine: *"I was 18 months old when she died. She was sick from birth and died at eight months of age. My dad turned off the machine and my mum never went to the cemetery. Later I tried to find her tomb but got lost".* Madeleine recognised that the pain she had in her body matched the little sister's deficient organs. The drawing (Figure 5.14) helped her bring the presence of her sister within her own psychic body. She identified with the sister who had a potential that had not developed. Early developmental aspects of Madeleine's personality had frozen in time, in a kind of symbiosis with the dead sister. I suggested to Madeleine that although the sister would always be present in her psyche, the sister's presence could take a different form. Madeleine chose to knit a bed to put her sister to rest.

I sensed fuzziness in my head and body and a lot of sadness at first that slowly ceded to clarity. The symbiosis between Madeleine's body and her sister's was being differentiated through the drawing, the knitting, and then the meaning-making. She was strong enough in herself to fully bring this very early memory that was frozen in time, and to be flooded by sensations and images that had been stored deep inside her body (Van der Kolk, 2014; Rothschild, 2000), and release the layers of the early family trauma, and loss of a child, a sister.

Conclusion

In the process of writing this chapter, I was carried by the bodily sensations, emotions, and images that Madeleine's artwork provoked in me at the time, enabling me to remember the experience of being with her in the space I was holding for both of us.

As our time together came to an end, Madeleine had planned another trip to France and had also been granted New Zealand citizenship. She said that she had reached her goals: being more secure within herself, grounded and con-nected in her senses, and connected to her children. She had broken the cycle of transgenerational trauma and was enjoying a more harmonious relationship with her husband. She felt empowered (an actor of her life) and purposeful (engaged in paid creative work). I experienced her as light, energetic, focused, confident, happy, and excited about her prospects. She remarked that she used to hate swimming, as the water reminded her of her mother, and was linked to amniotic fluid and her sadness. She had found a new love of being in the water. We reflected that *mère* (mother) and *mer* (sea) in French share the same sound.

Three years later, Madeleine asked for a catch-up session to let me know about her progress in life: she was still reaping the benefits of our time together and expressed gratitude for the process we had engaged in.

Acknowledgements

Thank you to Caroline Miller, our editor, for her patience, courage, inspira-tion, professionalism, hard work, unconditional support to me and to the com-munity of creative arts therapists in Aotearoa New Zealand.

Thank to my family, friends, and colleagues for their support and to my patients for their trust.

References

Abram, D. (1997). *The spell of the sensuous: Perception and language in a more-than-human world.* Vintage.

Amman, R. (1991). *Healing and transformation in sand play: Creative processes become visible.* Open Court.

Briere, J. N., & Scott, C. (2012). *Principles of trauma therapy: A guide to symptoms, evaluation and treatment.* Sage.

Carlson, R. J. (1979). The mother tongue in psychotherapy. *The Canadian Journal of Psychiatry, 24*, 542–546.

Cozolino, L. (2002). *The neuroscience of psychotherapy: Building and rebuilding the human.* W. W. Norton.

Cozolino, L. (2012). *The neuroscience of human relationships: Attachment and the developing social brain* (2nd ed.). W. W. Norton.

Dumas, G. (2011). Towards a two-body neuroscience. *Communicative and Integrative Biology, 4*, 349–352.

Erikson, E. H., & Erikson, J. M. (1998). *The life cycle completed (extended version).* W. W. Norton.

Freud, S. (1955, 2010). *The interpretation of dreams.* Basic Books.

Gendlin, E. T. (1998). *Focusing-oriented psychotherapy: A manual of the essential method.* Guilford Press.

Gerhardt, S. (2004). *Why love matters: How affection shapes the baby's brain.* Routledge.

Griner, D., & Smith, T. B. (2006). Culturally adapted mental health interventions: A meta-analytic review. *Psychotherapy: Theory, Research, Practice & Training, 43*, 531–548.

Halprin, D. (2005). *The expressive body in life, art and therapy: Working with movement, metaphor and meaning.* Jessica Kingsley.

Hass-Cohen, N., & Carr, R. (Eds.). (2008). *Art therapy and clinical neuroscience.* Jessica Kingsley.

Hass-Cohen, N. & Findlay, J. C. (2015). *Art therapy & the neuroscience of relationships, creativity, & resiliency skills and practices.* W.W. Norton.

Herman, J. L. 1992 (2015). *Trauma and recovery.* Basic Books.

Jung, C. G. (1997). *Man and his symbols.* Bantam Doubleday Dell.

Jung, C. G. (2003). *The spirit in man, art and literature.* Routledge.

Kabat-Zinn, J. (2005a). *Coming to our senses: Healing ourselves and the world through mindfulness.* Hyperion.

Kabat-Zinn, J. (2005b). *Wherever you go there you are: Mindfulness meditation in everyday life.* Hyperion.

Kalf, D. (2003). *Sandplay: A psychotherapeutic approach to the psyche.* Temenos Press.

Karen, R. (1998). *Becoming attached: First relationships and how they shape our capacity to love.* Oxford University.

Kempson, D., Conley, V. M., & Murdock, V. (2008). Unearthing the construct of transgenerational grief: The "ghost" of the sibling never known. *Illness, Crisis & Loss, 16*(4), 271–284. https://doi.org/10.2190/IL.16.4.aa

King, J. L. (2016). *Arts therapy, trauma, and neuroscience: Theoretical and practical perspectives.* Routledge.

Kurtz, R. (1990). *Body-centered psychotherapy: The Hakomi Method: The integrated use of mindfulness, nonviolence, and the body.* LifeRhythm.

Lecours, S., & Bouchard, M. (1997). Dimension of mentalisation: Outlining levels of psychic transformation. *The International Journal of Psychoanalysis, 78*(5), 855–875.

Levine, P. A. (2008). *Healing trauma: A pioneering program for restoring the wisdom of your body.* Sounds True.

Lieberman, M. D., Eisenberger, N. I., Crockett, M. J., Tom, S. M., Pfeifer, J. H., & Way, B. M. (2007). Putting feelings into words: Affect labelling disrupts amygdala activity in response to affective stimuli. *Psychological Science, 18*(5), 421–428.

Lightstone, J., & Suebert, A. (2009). The case of mistaken identity: Ego states and eating disorders. In R. Shapiro (Ed.), *EMDR solutions II.* W. W. Norton.

Malchiodi, C. A. (2002). *The soul's palette: Drawing on art's transformative powers for health and well-Being.* Shambhala.

Malchiodi, C. A. (2006). *Art therapy source book.* McGraw-Hill.

McNiff, S. (1992). *Art as medicine: Creating a therapy of the imagination.* Shambhala.

McWilliams, N. (2020). *Psychoanalytic diagnosis: Understanding personality structure in the clinical process* (2nd ed.). Guilford Press.

Mehling, W. E., Wrubel, J., Daubenmier, J. J., Price, C. J., Kerr, C. E., Silow, T., & Stewart, A. L. (2011). Body awareness: A phenomenological inquiry into the common ground of mind-body therapies. *Philosophy, Ethics, and Humanities in Medicine, 6,* Article ID 6.

Merleau-Ponty, M. (1962). *The phenomenology of perception.* Routledge and Kegan Paul.

Miller, C. (Ed.). (2014). *Assessment and outcomes in the arts therapies: A person-centred approach.* Jessica Kingsley.

Ogden, P., Minton, K., & Pain, C. (2006). *Trauma and the body: A sensory motor approach to psychotherapy.* W. W. Norton.

Pattis Zoja, E. (2004). *Sand play therapy: Treatment of psychopathologies.* Daimon Verlag.

Pearson, M., & Wilson, H. (2009). *Using expressive arts to work with mind, body and emotions.* Jessica Kingsley.

Perls, F. S. (1992). *Gestalt therapy verbatim.* The Gestalt Journal Press.

Perry, B. D., & Szalavitz, M. (2006). *The boy who was raised as a dog and other stories from a child psychiatrist's notebook: What traumatized children can teach us about loss, love, and healing.* Basic Books.

Pert, C. B. (1997). *Molecules of emotions: The science behind mind-body medicine.* Touchstone.

Porges, S. W. (2011). *The polyvagal theory: Neurophysiological foundations of emotions, attachment, communication, and self-regulation.* W. W. Norton.

Quatman, T. (2015). *Essential psychodynamic psychotherapy.* Routledge.

Robbins, A. (1994). *A multimodal approach to creative art therapy.* Jessica Kingsley.

Robbins, A. (2000). *The artist as therapist.* Jessica Kingsley.

Rothschild, B. (2000). *The body remembers: The psychophysiology of trauma and trauma treatment.* W. W. Norton.

Rothschild, B. (2017). *The body remembers Volume 2: Revolutionizing trauma treatment.* W. W. Norton.

Schmidt, S. J. (2009). *The developmental needs meeting strategy: An ego state therapy for healing adults with childhood trauma and attachment wounds.* DNMS Institute, LLC.

Schore, A. N. (1994). *Affect regulation and the origin of the self: The neurobiology of emotional development.* Lawrence Erlbaum Associates.

Schore, A. N. (2001). Effects of a secure attachment relationship on right brain development, affect regulation, and infant mental health. *Michigan Association for Infant Mental Health: Infant Mental Health Journal, 22*(1–2), 7–66.

Schore, A. N. (2007). Special section: Psychoanalytic research: Progress and process. Notes from Allan Schore's groups in developmental affective neuroscience and clinical practice. *Psychologist Psychoanalyst, XXVII*(1), 12–14.

Schore, A. N. (2012). *The science and the art of psychotherapy.* W. W. Norton.

Schore, A. N. (2019). *Right brain psychotherapy.* W. W. Norton.

Siegel, D. J. (2006). An interpersonal neurobiology approach to psychotherapy: Awareness, mirror neurons, and neural plasticity in the development of well-being. *Psychiatric Annals, 36*(4), 248–256.

Siegel, D. J. 2012 (2020). *The developing mind: How relationships and the brain interact to shape who we are* (3rd ed.). Guilford Press.

Stern, D. N. (2004). *The present moment: In psychotherapy and everyday life.* W. W. Norton.

Turner, B. A. (2005). *The handbook of sandplay therapy*. Temenos Press.

Van der Kolk, B. A. (2014). *The body keeps the score: Brain, mind, and body in the healing of trauma*. Viking.

Watkins, J. G., & Watkins, H. H. (1997). *Ego states: Theory and therapy*. W. W. Norton.

Weinrib, E. (2004). *Images of the self: The sand play therapy process*. Temenos Press.

Williams, M., Teasdale, J., Segal, Z., & Kabat-Zinn, J. (2007). *The mindful way through depression*. Guilford Press.

Winnicott, D. W. (2006). *Playing and reality* (first published in 1971). Routledge Classics.

6 We are here together for a while

Art therapy initiatives within a hospice setting in Singapore

Kim Hau Pang

Introduction

Singapore is a multi-ethnic and multicultural Asian society. Based on the last documented population census in 2010, the nation of 5 million consists of 74.1% Chinese, 13.4% Malay, 9.2% Indians, and 3.3% from other ethnic groups (Statistics Singapore, 2010). The concept of palliative care within such a demographic translates to a need for a culturally sensitive and inclusive approach and support.

This chapter is focused on three art therapy–informed initiatives within Assisi Hospice in Singapore, where the author serves as an art therapist. Art therapy can be contextualised for diverse population groups in a multitude of settings (Howie et al., 2013); and within the boundaries of this chapter, the context is palliative and bereavement care (Wood et al., 2019). These three initiatives, despite being independent of each other, provided a platform for other members of the interdisciplinary team to come alongside the art therapist to co-facilitate or support when necessary. This model of practice is also aligned with the "total pain, total care" clinical team–based approach prevalent within hospice settings (Hartley, 2014; Rubin, 2019).

In Singapore, emphasis is placed on the family as a basic unit of care. Social policies also draw on family-oriented values and cultures – such as the importance of family and kinship. Singaporeans are raised to be interdependent within the family unit (Peh & Ng, 2011). In the context of hospice/palliative care, this matches the perspective that family members and significant others are essentially 'invisible patients' for their role in the patient's life (Gross, 2014). What this means for psychosocial clinicians is that each patient engagement is considered and supported within the context of their families and their significant others.

In Singapore, the predecessors to the modern-day hospices were living spaces above Chinese funeral parlours. Located along Sago Lane (present-day Chinatown), these were named *death houses*. Banned by 1961, these were spaces where the locals were believed to be living their final days out (Thulaja, 2016). Little support was offered to the dying apart from shelter.

Singapore's first hospice, St. Joseph's Home, was opened in 1985 (The Straits Times, 1986) and a decade later, Singapore Hospice Council (SHC) was set up.

DOI: 10.4324/9781003082897-10

Art therapy services

Adopting an interdisciplinary team (IDT) approach, the art therapist works alongside a team of doctors, nurses, medical social workers, counsellors, pastoral care workers and other allied health therapists to care for each patient as a whole person (Assisi Hospice, n.d.). At present the art therapy service is available for inpatients and home-care and day-care patients.

The SHC defines hospice and palliative care as a holistic approach which focuses on pain and symptom control and improving quality of life through a team-based approach for both patients and their caregivers (Singapore Hospice Council, n.d.). Art therapy services at the hospice take place in groups or as individual engagement for patients and their significant others. Twice annually or on an as-needed basis, my art therapy colleague and I also plan art therapy directives to engage and support staff members through our staff welfare programme. This is aligned with our national guidelines for palliative care, whereby one of the domains of focus is the ability for staff members to reflect on their practice and express feelings related to their interactions with patients and their families (Duke NUS & Lien Centre for Palliative Care, 2011). The art therapists, with other members from the IDT, participate in the weekly journal club, sharing relevant clinical knowledge and skills for continuing development.

Art therapy services stretch across the whole continuum of hospice care services. The two art therapists have adopted a person-centred approach to art therapy for each of the service groups (Van Lith & Fenner, 2011). My art therapy colleague oversees the home care cases while my responsibility is the day-care art therapy programme. We also each have an individual inpatient caseload for art psychotherapy engagements. Within the context of the day-care centre, I work closely with my occupational therapy colleague in the planning of groups to engage the day-care patients. The art therapy groups which I am overseeing fall loosely between "art making with emphasis on skill development and mastery" and "programme facilitated and structured art groups" within the continuum of practice (Van Lith & Fenner, 2011; Figure 6.1). Clinical goals may be realised in the learning of an art skill through a curriculum

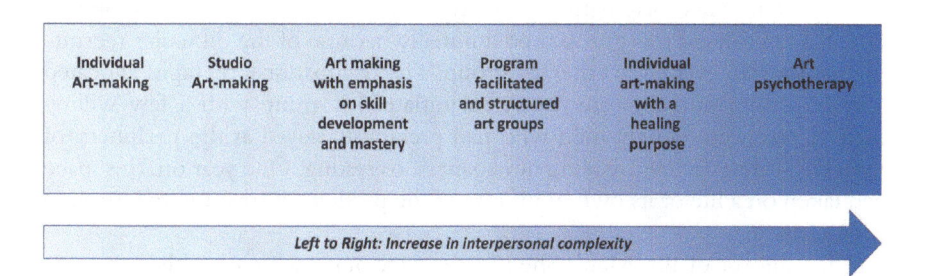

Figure 6.1 The continuum of practice (Van Lith & Fenner, 2011)

and in broad personal expressions which may result in an exhibition, project, or showcase occasionally.

Art therapy group

There is still life

There are two art therapy groups in the day-care centre programme. Participants for these groups are mostly referred by the day-care manager or the occupational therapist based on the participant's indication of interest from the list of programmes our day-care centre is offering. This once-a-week art therapy group focuses on a semi-structured theme-based approach, whereby familiar subjects such as fruits, flowers, or vegetables are brought in for still-life drawings. Each participant is given a range of wet and dry medium to work with. Innovative and personalised artmaking methods have arisen from the participants themselves and shared within the group amongst others over the weeks. The creative environment resembles a 'structured open studio' where participants, staff, and trained volunteers socialise with artmaking oscillating between the foreground and the background for an hour each week. In recent months, some of the artwork done by these participants has also been selected, with their given consent, to be used for fundraising merchandise for the hospice. This gives an added dimension to the level of contribution they can be a part of, instead of being only a recipient of palliative health care services and it has effectively allowed others a glimpse into the vibrancy of the lives of these individuals. This art group also serves as a space occasionally where medical social worker colleagues from the Psychosocial Services (PSS) department join in the session to spend time creating alongside the participants and getting to know them better.

Men united

An adapted Men's Shed model for a hospice setting

The other art therapy group is a men's focused group modelled after the community Men's Shed originating from Australia (Moylan et al., 2013; Golding, 2015). I considered this group model initially because of the difficulty recruiting men for the weekly art therapy group. The occupational therapist allocated a space within our day-care centre to initiate this group with a few willing men. These were elderly men who had previously stayed at the periphery of most day-care activities, reading newspapers, or resting. One year on, this space had taken on a life of its own, with one of the participants naming the group – Men United.

The concept of the Men's Shed is a service approach to health care, providing male-friendly spaces in the community where men can connect with each other while having opportunities to learn practical skills and develop new interests (Australian Men's Shed Association, 2017). The aim of the Men's Shed is to improve the mental health and social well-being of men, by providing a casual space in which men interact. Spaces provide company, specific working spaces for projects, social space to reduce isolation, and accessibility to health care (in this case being sited within a palliative health care facility). They have a casual approach with a lack of compulsion which promotes learning and well-being, being part of something bigger, to be able to continue giving back and feeling useful, and a place to develop a sense of community with a safe space to be vulnerable in the company of other men. For some, just having a fixed time and space provided a routine that resembles a similar sense of employment-like satisfaction, and for others, having a regular place to go to with no obligations gives them a reason to leave the house (Kelly et al., 2019; Moylan et al., 2013; Wilson & Cordier, 2013).

Initiating the shed

The concept of having an allocated handiwork area at home is uncommon in Singapore's context due to the limited floor area in most living spaces. According to Müller (2020), about 91% of the local population live in apartment flats built by the Housing Developmental Board of Singapore as of 2018. This means that most individuals do not have the space for handiwork at home. The programming and setup for the shed takes reference from studies published from Australia, Canada, Ireland, and the United Kingdom (Moylan et al., 2013; Mackenzie et al., 2017; Lefkowich & Richardson, 2016; Kelly et al., 2019). I oversee the weekly running of the shed with assistance from two therapy aides. The shed now provides a regular daily group for male day-care patients as a social workspace, with a shared work area taking central dominance. The absence of a structured programme facilitated self-directed approaches to utilise the area. In the middle of the designated space is a simple layout of the work area and adjacent to it is a shelf for materials and basic tools. Beside the work area are chairs where they can choose to sit should they not want to use the workspace. One of the members built a traditional Malay house based on his childhood home. Others adapted wooden clothes pegs to make other items and worked with Paulownia wood, while one member did a series of drawings to remember and revisit his childhood memories. The space is also used by individuals who wish to be working on more guided projects, which also allows men to provide mentorship to new participants. There is a selection of hand tools such as a range of handsaws, carpenter's square, an assortment of clamps, small bench vices, and adhesives for wood, with a small additional range of power tools.

In the shed

A 74-year-old Malay man, Mr M, is a regular attendee of the shed. He started fishing to help family expenses on a sampan – a traditional flat-bottomed

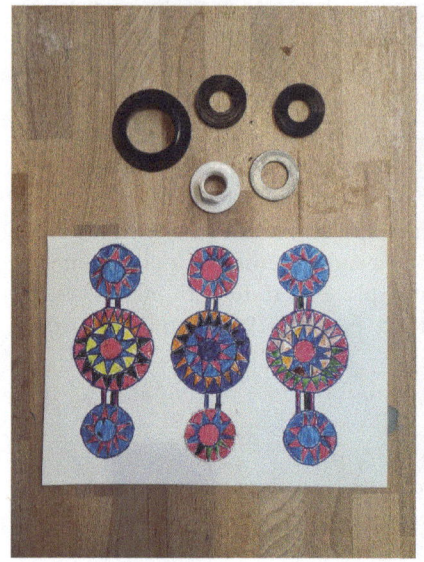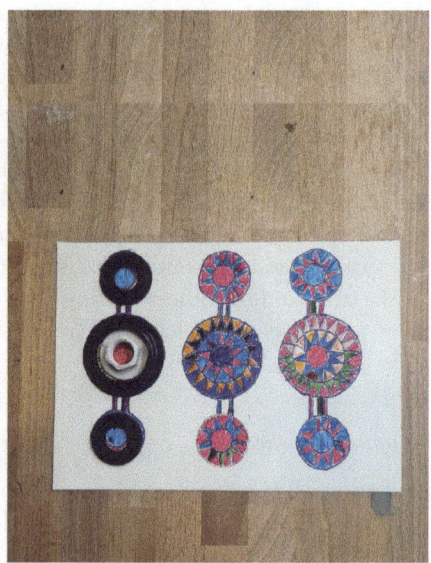

Figure 6.2 Mr M.'s found objects: stencil and bicycle gear drawing (2020)

Malay wooden boat used for fishing. From the age of 12, he lived on the sampan, under the stars without a roof over his head. When he comes to the shed, he works on his own drawings or spends time socialising with others. His choice of working with dry medium traces back to his preference for predictability and control, a luxury he did not have over his environment and life for many years. Over the weeks while witnessing his artmaking process, he started to share with me his collection of drawing stencils made of primarily found objects that he salvages from his living environment (Figure 6.2). The casual approach in the shed effectively created an open space for Mr M to engage at his own pace in a safe environment where he felt accepted.

The shed has evolved into a community and a holding space where staff can break news of other participants' passing to those who were close to them. On one occasion as we broke the news of the losses of three members, one of the therapy aides led these men in Al-Fātiḥah – a culturally specific prayer offered for each of the demised individually by name. In reference to Perry's model (2006, p. 41), the limbic and cortical systems are associated with the development and regulation of emotional states that relate to play and creative activities involving mark-making, symbolism, pretence, and social interaction. These engagements will allow the systems in the brainstem to facilitate regulation through helping clients 'feel safe within therapy through therapeutic containment and the establishment of boundaries' (Perry, 2006, p. 41; cited by Donnelly, 2017, p. 146).

The men's shed gives these men the environment to reprise their role as providers and contributors towards society, in the company of other men. It allows staff to get to know the men and normalise their experiences as individuals with life-limiting illnesses while remembering those who were once with them. Providing this space also provides a place of considerable safety and creativity for these men experiencing grief and loss towards the end of their own lives.

Always Remembering Them (ART)

Art and bereavement

Art is an effective tool when words alone are deemed inadequate to support the exploration and expression of emotionally charged areas, like bereavement. Through the process of making an artwork, an individual can experience the reconnecting of bonds that were "severed through loss" (Dreifuss-Kattan, 2016, p. 2). Losses are experienced beyond the constraints of time and space. Often the process of grieving involves a need to find a form of psychological balance. This would mean that to make sense of the present loss, a bereaved individual not only mourns in the here and now but will also revisit earlier losses at the same time. Through giving a form to this experience by means of visualisation, artmaking can stabilise the self and re-establish the balance after the loss. This is often achieved through the internal and external dialogue an individual goes through during the artmaking process (Bat-Or & Garti, 2019). Artmaking is a channel of release for these intense emotions related to loss by these bereaved individuals (Davis, 1989). The art medium in this context facilitates the containment of both conscious and unconscious content pertaining to losses both past and present (Dreifuss-Kattan, 2016). The artwork created by the bereaved individual will hence serve to memorialise their relationship with those who have departed (Potash & Handel, 2012). One such example is *Repetition Nineteen III* (Hesse, 1968) by the late American sculptor Eva Hesse. The random placement of knee-high, irregular receptacles in the room led to an association to departed souls – drawing direct reference to Hesse's "traumatic and painful losses within her immediate family" (Dreifuss-Kattan, 2016, p. 114).

Within the multidisciplinary team, art therapists attend weekly departmental rounds during which we actively contribute and plan goals of care and relevant art therapy interventions alongside the medical social workers and counsellors for each case. This close working relationship contributed to art therapy coming alongside the Psychological Support Service in supporting the Inter-Faith Memorial Service (IFMS) held at the hospice tri-annually, for experiences of individual loss to be heard and acknowledged (Rollo-Carlson, 2016). This forms the background for ART.

ART is conceptualised as a safe open-and-facilitated art space within the hospice setting for clinical and non-clinical staff. Working constantly with people experiencing grief and loss can lead to heightened stress reactions and difficulties with emotional regulation. Malchiodi (2020) describes regulation as "ways to manage and release stress, including how we cope with sadness" (p. 1). These reactions share some characteristics with the impact of various forms of trauma on the brain and body. Art therapy when applied to this context is known to facilitate self-regulation, and this becomes one of the reasons it is often applied to assist in the reduction of "hyperactivation and stress responses that result from traumatic events", for both adults and children (Malchiodi, 2020, p. 1). ART's intention is to allow individual expression of personal grief and loss within a safe and non-judgemental environment. To maintain a sense of openness, an open studio approach has been adopted to facilitate this initiative (Moon, 2016).

This space opens from 09:00 to 17:00 hours to accommodate staff on shifts or with breaks during the day. Individuals may drop in at any point in time to make art or drop in and pick up art materials they might need to work on in their own space. Members from the PSS team and both the art therapists take turns being present in the room to provide a safe holding environment as an added layer of support for the bereaved individuals. Drawing reference to the client–art axis of the therapeutic triangle (Schaverien, 2000), the therapeutic emphasis of this initiative lies in allowing the artmaking process to be the healing agent (Bat-Or & Garti, 2019). As such, there is no facilitated discussion and processing of personal artwork. Each staff member who participates in ART can give a title to their artwork and a 30-word statement to give a voice to their work if they wish. They may also give consent for the artwork to be part of the exhibition during the IFMS possibly as an 'anonymous artist'. Ultimately, the artwork is the property of the individual creating it (ATCB, 2019) so they have the final say about what is done with it.

IFMS

This annual service honours the various beliefs and cultural customs of the Singapore society and provides a continuation of support for families and significant others following the death of a patient (Bardot, 2013; Singapore Hospice Council, 2018). This is a time where religious leaders from different faiths gather to remember and honour the sacred lives of those who have departed. This is also a space where bereaved persons get to meet and speak with fellow bereaved individuals alongside the staff members and volunteers of the hospice who have been a part of this journey. Having the artworks created for ART sited at the common area where people gather provides validation of the grief and pain, each contained in the individual artwork without any exchange of words needed. Some of these works serve as conversation starters and some as backdrops reflecting and honouring memories with reassurance. The presentation of the works as a single exhibition within the IFMS also hint at the universality and individuality of grief and of our shared humanity and mortality as we remember those who have departed. This collective experience serves as a reminder that grief and love are but different sides of the same coin (Shear, 2016).

Effects of community and social engagements

For the patients in the hospice

The notion of community and togetherness is a strong underlying concept in hospice care. The focus on the different aspects of pain a dying individual might be experiencing – physically, psychologically, socially, and spiritually requires a team approach (Saunders & Baines, 1983). Beginning with the clinicians, this sense of community extends outwards to the art therapy programme provided for the individuals and their significant others, and to our colleagues at the hospice. Art therapy, being a low-intensity and low-cost intervention, is often observed to be delivered within nursing homes and community environments to support such needs (Roswiyani et al., 2017). There is growing evidence supporting social engagement as helping individuals maintain mental fitness (GCBH, 2017). Through the artmaking process within the art therapy group, older adult patients will be engaged through a combination of visual, emotional, and behavioural outputs that integrate cognitive and relational elements. This helps them externalise and further define their individual experiences (King et al., 2019).

Positive outcomes in cognitive functioning have also been associated with social relationships for older adults (Kelly et al., 2017) and group-based approaches provide a safe environment to promote such connections. The experience of safety is a need to be considered at the beginning of any therapeutic process as it is vital in the facilitation of a client's "engagement and healing" (Prendiville, 2017, p. 8). This sense of safety and familiarity is one of the primary considerations while setting up the Men's Shed. The establishment of a gender-specific safe space for self-directed or supported 'play' has been a success. The men have been spotted lounging in that area for longer hours, socialising in between activities and even during mealtimes after clearing up the workspace. Some of them also started showcasing works they have completed in the area as an extension of their presence and ownership in that space.

Yalom (1995) wrote about the benefits of group approaches. He noted that feelings of isolation through the sharing of a common experience will diminish with groups, allowing individuals to connect with others who have experienced similar challenges. Mirror neurons come into play within group and individual settings, giving rise to empathy for the self and towards others (Wilson, 2014). Having these social engagements and support with other like-minded individuals promotes resilience against stress, which may be different from participating in social activities with family members (Ozbay et al., 2007). This describes the intention for both the art therapy group and Men United in providing a space, through a shared interest of creative expression or a gender-specific programme to facilitate meaningful relationships and social engagements.

For the staff in the hospice

The application of art within the context of the staff support programme ART has provided a social and personal lens to dying and grief, as grief is a universal experience, not a disease or a condition to be treated (Barrington, 2008; Horwitz & Wakefield, 2007; Valentine, 2008). The normalisation and validation of individual experiences and emotional states are two of the direct applications of neuroscience to art therapy practices (King et al., 2019). A study in Hong Kong (Potash et al., 2014) reflected that an art therapy–based approach had helped palliative care workers come to terms with inner conflicts in a safe and supportive environment. The loss of a loved one, a relationship, or an identity equates to the symbolic loss of oneself. Counsellors would describe this process of loss as "falling apart or to pieces" (Arnason, 2007). Through this, grief can be understood as a response towards this breaking and dissolving of social and intimate relationships. It is a painful reconstruction of the individual's everyday life (Bradbury, 1999). Charmaz and Milligan (2006, p. 525) suggested that grief is seen as an interpersonal process emerging from relationships, attachments, expectations, and obligations. Social and cultural influences have a role in grief responses, making experiences of grief and loss personal and highly subjective.

Freud (1957) looked at grief work as a continuous process where an individual focuses on the lost object. Bion (1962) wrote about how grief is an attempt to live with the loss while finding ways to symbolise it and process it psychologically. When an individual is grieving, imagination fills the void, "replacing absence and emptiness with new memories and imagery, which in turn engender creativity" (Dreifuss-Kattan, 2016, p. 3). In essence, the arts are "neuropsychology in action" (Zaidel, as cited in King et al., 2019, p. 149). What artmaking provides is an integration of experiences for developmental growth. Verbal modes of therapy alone will not lead to full recovery. Changes in the brainstem and midbrain cannot be reached by talking alone. When recalling both early and disturbing memories, the right hemisphere of the human brain is predominantly activated (Prendiville, 2017; Van der Kolk, 2015). This suggests that activities engaging the right brain would be necessary in the processing of unresolved trauma and the modification of "embodied and implicit memories" (Prendiville, 2017, p. 8). Artmaking's reparative ability through harnessing imagination by means of visual expression harmonises memories with new perceptions and the gradual regulation of affect aids in the personal reconstruction of meaning through witnessing one's own creation. This facilitates an important psychological change for finding meaning in a world altered by loss, as the ability to make sense of it is identified as a key factor for successful adaptation to losses (Neimeyer, 2001; Wilson et al., 2016). Through the sharing with others, such as the presentation of the artworks at the ART exhibition, the internal witness is strengthened and gradually the newly expressed perception will substitute for the actual loss, allowing for the reintegration of the self (Dreifuss-Kattan, 2016).

Embarking on the process of making an artwork, the individual goes through a process of self-reflection and knowing (Allen, 1995). The artwork, a physical manifestation of this knowing functions as both the subject and object of reflection, allowing individuals to find the thread through the past and the present (Grushka, 2005). Embedded within these artworks are "numinous or spirit-filled" images, signposts reflecting into the depths of oneself (Allen, 1995, p. 87). Such reflective practices may seem uncommon within a medical setting, but with individual and cultural differences becoming part of medical education, there is a recognition that both disciplines of medicine and humanities share a similar subject of focus on the human experience (Gordon, 2005; Ong & Anantham, 2019).

Conclusion

We are here together, for a while only

Endings and terminations are an inevitable part of our everyday experiences outside our control and sometimes 'without comment' (Edwards, 1997, p. 49). These are human uncertainties (Gordon, 2005). Art therapy is recognised as an effective way to support individuals through different life transitions and experiences when words become difficult. The arts therapies have been applied and integrated into palliative and bereavement care internationally (Bardot, 2008; Bat-Or & Garti, 2019; Wood et al., 2019). On an intrapersonal level, artmaking is also recognised as an effective therapeutic approach to mirror and attend to an individual's inner experiences of grief and loss (Dreifuss-Kattan, 2016; Pang, 2018, 2021; Rollo-Carlson, 2016).

Serving as an art therapist within a setting where service recipients are individuals with life-limiting conditions put me in a position of privilege to be journeying with families during this important chapter of their lives. On occasions, we also bear witness to similar chapters in the lives of our colleagues. The arts therapies allow the unique narratives of each individual to be understood from their personal and social experiences within a person-centred relationship (Ong & Anantham, 2019). The group-based art therapy approaches outlined in this chapter provide support.

Art therapy as part of the interdisciplinary care in a hospice provides an additional layer of support for the body, mind, and spirit of individuals. The communication of emotions, mood elevation, and connecting to self and to others, are some tangible benefits art therapy can bring (Buday, 2013). These initiatives have supported the creativity of individuals and the way they heal through the establishment of a safe environment where an "interplay can take place" (McNiff, 2004, p. 51). As a human service profession, art therapy with other health care disciplines has an important role in the hospice environment to relieve and to comfort. After all, we are only here on this earth for a while so let us cherish each other's humanity as we continue to serve alongside one another together.

Acknowledgements

To all my patients, thank you for being the best teachers I can dream of having as a clinician and, most important, as a fellow human being.

And to my parents for guiding me forward despite your departures so that I can better serve others through the losses in my own life.

References

Allen, P. B. (1995). *Art is a way of knowing*. Shambhala.

Arnason, A. (2007). Fall apart and put yourself back together again: The anthropology of death and bereavement counselling in Britain. *Mortality*, *12*(1), 48–65.

Assisi Hospice. (n.d.). *About us. Assisi hospice*. www.assisihospice.org.sg/about-us/#ourhistory

ATCB. (2019). *Code of ethics: Conduct and disciplinary procedure*. www.atcb.org/Ethics/ATCBCode

Australian Men's Shed Association. (2017). *What Is a Men's Shed?* https://mensshed.org/what-is-a-mens-shed/

Bardot, H. (2008). Expressing the inexpressible: The resilient healing of a client and the art therapist. *Art Therapy: Journal of the American Art Therapy Association*, *25*(4), 183–186.

Bardot, H. (2013). The universality of grief and loss. In P. Howie, S. Prasad, & J. Kristel (Eds.), *Using art therapy with diverse populations crossing cultures and abilities* (pp. 256–266). Jessica Kingsley.

Barrington, C. A. (2008). *Exploring the nature and meaning of art with older adults in hospice* (Master's dissertation). Florida State University. http://diginole.lib.fsu.edu/etd

Bat-Or, M., & Garti, D. (2019). Art therapist's perceptions of the role of the art medium in the treatment of bereaved clients in art therapy. *Death Studies*, *43*(3), 193–203.

Bion, W. R. (1962). *Learning from experience*. Maresfield.

Bradbury, M. (1999). *Representations of death: A social psychological perspective*. Routledge.

Buday, K. M. (2013). Engage, empower, and enlighten: Art therapy and image making in hospice care. *Progress in Palliative Care*, *21*(2), 83–88.

Charmaz, K., & Milligan, M. J. (2006). Grief. In J. E. Stets & J. H. Turner (Eds.), *Handbook of the sociology of emotions* (pp. 516–543). Springer.

Davis, C. B. (1989). The use of art therapy and group process with grieving children. *Issues in Comprehensive Paediatric Nursing*, *12*(4), 269–280.

Donnelly, C. C. (2017). The healing power of images. In E. Prendiville & J. Howard (Eds.), *Creative Psychotherapy* (p. 146). Routledge.

Dreifuss-Kattan, E. (2016). *Art and mourning: The role of creativity in healing trauma and loss*. Routledge.

Duke NUS & Lien Centre for Palliative Care. (2011, October 4). *Report on the national strategy for palliative care*. https://singaporehospice.org.sg/site2019/wp-content/uploads/Report_on_National_Strategy_for_Palliative_Care-5Jan2012.pdf

Edwards, D. (1997). Endings. *Inscape*, *2*(2), 49–56.

Freud, S. (1957). *Mourning and melancholia. Standard edition of the complete work of Sigmund Freud*. Hogarth Press.

GCBH. (2017). *The brain and social connectedness: GCBH recommendations on social engagement and brain health*. www.aarp.org/content/dam/aarp/health/brain_health/2017/02/gcbh-social-engagement-report.pdf

Golding, B. (Ed.). (2015). *The men's shed movement: The company of men*. Common Ground Publishing.

Gordon, J. (2005). Medical humanities: To cure sometimes, to relieve often, to comfort always. *The Medical Journal of Australia, 182*(1), 5–8.

Gross, J. (2014, November 17). *Seeing the 'invisible patient'*. https://newoldage.blogs.nytimes.com/2014/11/17/seeing-the-invisible-patient/

Grushka, K. (2005). Artists as reflective self-learners and cultural communicators: An exploration of the qualitative aesthetic dimension of knowing self through reflective practice in art-making. *Reflective Practice, 6*(3), 353–366.

Hartley, N. (2014). The model and philosophy of hospice and end of life care. In N. Hartley (Ed.), *End of life care: A guide for therapists, artists and arts therapists* (pp. 29–50). Jessica Kingsley.

Hesse, E. (1968). *Repetition nineteen III*. https://www.moma.org/collection/works/81930

Horwitz, A. V., & Wakefield, J. C. (2007). *The loss of sadness. How psychiatry transformed normal sorrow into depressive disorder*. Oxford University Press.

Howie, P., Prasad, S., & Kristel, J. (Eds.). (2013). *Using art therapy with diverse populations: Crossing cultures and abilities*. Jessica Kingsley.

Jakoby, N. R. (2012). Grief as a social emotion: Theoretical perspectives. *Death Studies, 36*(8), 679–711.

Kelly, D., Steiner, A., Mason, H., & Teasdale, S. (2019). Men's sheds: A conceptual exploration of the causal pathways for health and well-being. *Health & Social Care in the Community, 27(5)*, 1147–1157.

Kelly, M., Duff, H., Kelly, S., McHugh Power, J., Brennan, S., Lawlor, B., & Loughrey, D. (2017). The impact of social activities, social networks, social support and social relationships on the cognitive functioning of healthy older adults: A systematic review. *Systematic Reviews, 6*(1), 1–18.

King, J. L., Kaimal, G., Konopka, L., Belkofer, C., & Strang, C. E. (2019). Practical applications of neuroscience-informed art therapy. *Art Therapy, 36*(3), 149–156.

Lefkowich, M., & Richardson, N. (2016). Men's health in alternative spaces: Exploring men's shed in Ireland. *Health Promotion International, 11*(1), 1–11.

Mackenzie, C. S., Roger, K., Robertson, S., Oliffe, J. L., Nurmi, M. A., & Urquhart, J. (2017). Counter and complicit masculine discourse among men's shed members. *American Journal of Men's Health, 11*(4), 1224–1236.

Malchiodi, C. (2020). Trauma, self-regulation, and expressive arts therapy. *Psychology Today (Therapy)*, 1–3.

McNiff, S. (2004). *Art heals: How creativity cures the soul*. Shambhala.

Moon, C. H. (2016). Open studio approach to art therapy. In D. E. Gussak & M. L. Rosal (Eds.), *The Wiley handbook of art therapy* (pp. 112–121). John Wiley & Sons Ltd.

Moylan, M. M., Carey, L. B., Blackburn, R., Hayes, R., & Robinson, P. (2013). The men's shed: Providing biopsychosocial and spiritual support. *Journal of Religion and Health, 54*(1), 221–234.

Müller, J. (2020). *Home ownership rate in Singapore 2009–2018*. www.statista.com/statistics/664518/home-ownership-rate-singapore/

Neimeyer, R. A. (Ed.). (2001). *Meaning reconstruction and the experience of loss*. American Psychological Association.

Ong, E. K., & Anantham, D. (2019). The medical humanities: Reconnecting with the soul of medicine. *The Annals, Academy of Medicine, Singapore, 48*(7), 233–237.

Ozbay, F., Johnson, D. C., Dimoulas, E., Morgan, C. A., Charney, D., & Southwick, S. (2007). Social support and resilience to stress: From neurobiology to clinical practice. *Psychiatry (Edgmont), 4*(5), 35–40.

Pang, K. H. (2018). 'From dusk till dawn': Finding healing through creative expressions. *Australian and New Zealand Journal of Arts Therapy*, *13*(1 & 2), 131–136.

Pang, K. H. (2021). The aftermath of losing mum and dad: Grieving through creative expression with everyday objects. In D. Wong & R. Lay (Eds.), *Found objects in art therapy: Materials and process* (pp. 151–164). Jessica Kingsley.

Peh, C. W., & Ng, T. W. (2011). Palliative social work in Singapore. In T. Altilio & S. Otis-Green (Eds.), *Oxford textbook of palliative social work* (pp. 579–585). Oxford University Press.

Perry, B. D. (2006). The neurosequential model of therapeutics: Applying principles of neuroscience to clinical work with traumatized and maltreated children, (p. 41). In N. B. Webb (Ed.), *Working with traumatized youth in child welfare* (pp. 27–52). Guilford Press.

Potash, J. S., & Handel, S. (2012). Memory boxes. In R. Neimeyer (Ed.), *Techniques in grief therapy: Creative strategies for counselling the bereaved* (pp. 263–266). Routledge.

Potash, J., S., Y. Ho, A. H., Chan, F., Wang, X., Lu, W., & Cheng, C. (2014). Can art therapy reduce death anxiety and burnout in end-of-life care workers? A quasi-experimental study. *International Journal of Palliative Nursing*, *20*(5), 233–240.

Prendiville, E. (2017). Neurobiology for psychotherapists. In E. Prendiville & J. Howard (Eds.), *Creative psychotherapy: Applying the principles of neurobiology to play and expressive arts-based practice* (pp. 7–20). Routledge.

Rollo-Carlson, C. (2016). Thawing frozen grief. In R. A. Neimeyer (Ed.), *Techniques of grief therapy: Assessment and interventions* (pp. 209–211). Routledge and Taylor & Francis Group.

Roswiyani, R., Kwakkenbos, L., Spijker, J., & Witteman, C. (2017). The effectiveness of combining visual art activities and physical exercise for older adults on well-being or quality of life and mood: A scoping review. *Journal of Applied Gerontology*, *38*(12), 1784–1804.

Rubin, S. Y. (2019). An art therapist's approach to total pain. In M. J. M. Woods, B. Jacobson, & H. Cridford (Eds.), *The international handbook of art therapy in palliative and bereavement care* (pp. 215–231). Routledge.

Saunders, C., & Baines, M. (1983). *Living with dying: The management of terminal disease.* Oxford University Press.

Schaverien, J. (2000). The triangular relationship and the aesthetic countertransferences in analytical art psychotherapy. In A. Gilroy & G. McNeilly (Eds.), *The changing shape of art therapy: New developments in theory and practice* (pp. 55–83). Jessica Kingsley.

Shear, M. K. (2016). Grief is a form of love. In R. A. Neimeyer (Ed.), *Techniques of grief therapy: Assessment and interventions* (pp. 14–18). Routledge and Taylor & Francis Group.

Singapore Hospice Council. (n.d.). *Palliative care overview. Singapore hospice council.* https://singaporehospice.org.sg/palliativecare/

Singapore Hospice Council. (2018, June–August 14–15). Manoeuvring grief and bereavement in palliative care. *The Hospice Link.* https://singaporehospice.org.sg/hospice-link/

Statistics Singapore. (2010). *Census of population, 2010: Advance census release.* www.singstat.gov.sg/pubn/popn/C2010acr.pdf

The Straits Times. (1986). In Singapore, a place to die peacefully. *The Straits Times.* https://eresources.nlb.gov.sg/newspapers/Digitised/Article/straitstimes19860701-1.2.67.3

Thulaja, N. R. (2016). *Sago lane, national library board.* https://eresources.nlb.gov.sg/infopedia/articles/SIP_299_2005-01-11.html

Valentine, C. (2008). *Bereavement narratives: Continuing bonds in the 21st century.* Routledge.

Van der Kolk, B. (2015). *The body keeps the score: Brain, mind, and body in the healing of trauma.* Penguin Books.

Van Lith, T., & Fenner, P. (2011). The practice continuum: Conceptualizing a person-centred approach to art therapy. *Australian and New Zealand Journal of Arts Therapy, 6*(1), 17–22.

Wilson, N. J., & Cordier, R. (2013). A narrative review of Men's Sheds literature: Reducing social isolation and promoting men's health and well-being. *Health & Social Care in the Community, 21*(5), 451–463.

Wilson, N. J., James, H., & Gabriel, L. (2016). Making sense of loss and grief: The value of in-depth assessments. *Bereavement Care, 35*(2), 67–77.

Wilson, R. Z. (2014). *Neuroscience for counsellors. Practical applications for counsellors,* Jessica Kingsley.

Wood, M. J. M., Jacobson, B., & Cridford, H. (Eds.). (2019). *The international handbook of art therapy in palliative and bereavement care.* Routledge.

Yalom, I. D. (1995). *The theory and practice of group psychotherapy.* Basic Books.

7 Imagination and art therapy

A bridge to transformation for traumatised clients

Mariana Torkington

Introduction

The experience of artmaking in the context of the therapeutic alliance places clients at the centre of their own trajectory in the presence of the therapist who acts as a witness and co-creator. Rubin (1999) refers to the necessary conditions for therapy and states that it is the responsibility of the therapist to establish a framework for freedom (p. 140). Such conditions encompass physical as well as psychological aspects. According to Rubin (1999) "psychodynamic psychotherapists have been especially attracted to the use of art in their work because of the ability of imagery to bypass defences" (p. 73). Wadeson (1980 as cited in Rubin, 2001, p. 306) states that "whatever happens in art therapy happens within the container of the relationship." Integral to this process with clients is respect for and trust in the imagery as carrying the potential for insight and transformation. Another important principle in the context of art therapy practice is the triangular relationship involving the client, the therapist, and the art process and product, through engagement in meaningful and interactive dialogue with the art and in verbal exchanges.

The field of art therapy is predicated on the belief that the "creative process involved in the making of art is healing and life-enhancing" (Moon, 2002, p. 306). This is supported by a range of theoretical frameworks. In recent decades, neuroscience has acknowledged the benefits of engaging imagination in the treatment of trauma and contributed to these discussions as well. According to Kapitan (2010), the field of neuroscience is developing ideas about empathy, learning and consciousness and posits that "mental processes in art therapy derive from brain activity" (p. 158). Kapitan (2010) suggests that "art therapy exerts its healing effects by inducing new learning at the structural level of the brain that is in a constant state of becoming" (p. 158). In this context, imagination plays a vital role in art therapy and in brain development. Perry (2008, as cited in Kapitan, 2010, p. 158) asserts that art therapy supports changes to brain structure and assists to build new networks through imaging, patterning, somatic sensory cues, touch, and movement.

According to Rubin (2001, p. 319) "imagination represents a state of consciousness where the different elements in a situation can meet, influence one

DOI: 10.4324/9781003082897-11

another, and create new patterns of interaction". Jung developed a therapeutic method for personal healing that relies on the use of imagination. He termed this approach to working with images of his unconscious, 'active imagination'.

Chodorow (2006, as cited in Papadopoulos, pp. 215–216) referred to this process as

> turning attention and curiosity toward the inner world of the imagination and expressing it symbolically, all the while seeking a self-reflective, psychological point of view. The many creative forms of active imagination include visions in the mind's eye, hypnagogic images that float up not only as visual impressions, but also auditory images, motor images and other somatosensory impressions; dialogue with inner figures; expressing the imagination through any, or all of the arts, the symbolic enactment of Sandplay and many others.

Jung introduced universal patterns and images that he referred to as archetypes and described these in terms of modes of functioning. He saw 'the archetype-as-such' as the inherent neuropsychic system, responsible for patterns of behaviour in our environment (Stevens, 1982, p. 18).

Contemporary arts therapists have embraced theories from psychoanalytic literature, Jung's depth psychology, gestalt art therapy, and integrative art therapy (Hogan, 2015) to try to clarify what takes place in the therapist's interactions with clients. Developments in neuroscience and neuroplasticity have contributed to this discussion in recent decades.

According to the British Association of Art Therapists (BAAT, 2020) art therapy is a form of psychotherapy that uses art media as its primary mode of expression and communication. Through the act of creating art and reflecting on the process and the medium, individuals can increase self-awareness and develop resilience. Exploring the links between neuroscience and art therapy has also been at the forefront of journal articles and BAAT conferences, such as its inaugural conference exploring brain research and implicit memory.

Franklin's (2010) study of mirror neurons "underscores how observing an art creation causes subtle, neural-level changes in the observer that mirror the feelings of the creator" (as cited in Klorer, 2017, p. 12) stimulating an empathic exchange. McNamee (2003, 2006) studied bilateral art activity and suggested that "clients engaged in bilateral art activities use both hands in an effort to stimulate the memories and experiences that reside in both sides of the brain (2003, p. 284). It is presumed that this helps with systemic reprocessing and integration. Hass-Cohen and Findlay (2015) developed the art therapy relational neuroscience model informed by principles of relationships. Studies such as these have signalled the relationship between art creation, which employs the imagination, and the development of neural pathways and empathic exchanges, which serve to nurture deeper communication and enhance treatment recovery.

Flora's art therapy

In this section, I introduce an adolescent client who was 13 years old when she was first referred for art therapy by her social worker. Flora had a background of early childhood trauma. She came from a large family of African ancestry and was separated from her parents and her siblings, who were dispersed across the city where she resided. Flora was in foster care herself when she commenced therapy. Funding was secured through Accident Compensation Corporation (ACC), a government department that offers fully or partly funded integrated therapy services following sexual and other traumatic events experienced in New Zealand. The ACC can provide long-term counselling and psychotherapy services for clients who meet their criteria. At the time of the referral, Flora had been exposed to inappropriate sexual behaviour by a male who was unknown to her. Flora's therapy took place over a period of 18 months.

An assessment was conducted in the first few sessions and incorporated the use of the Outcome Ratings Scale (ORS; Miller et al., 2003) to attempt to gain insight into Flora's self-perception. Flora's presentation in the early stages of therapy provided some insight into her attachment difficulties. Flora was cautious and withdrawn. During the initial interview, it was reported that she was often tearful and dissociative, appearing to block things out. Flora herself reported that she had scary thoughts and was feeling stressed. While she presented with low self-esteem and a lack of confidence, there was a marked difference in her presentation when she handled art materials. She was comfortable working with art materials, and her caregiver reported that art provided her with hours of enjoyment at home.

During the assessment process, Flora articulated that she wanted to work on being brave. Gathering information in the assessment phase is an important task as it helps to clarify issues and build a clearer picture of the work that lies ahead. Miller (2014) stated that assessment can be wide ranging, can be informed by various therapeutic approaches, and can be influenced by client goals. Miller (2014) asserts that there has been a shift in the arts therapies towards assessments that utilise "a more subjective approach in terms of capturing the experience of the client and working with this, rather than relying on therapist interpretation" (p. 18). The Child Outcome Rating Scale (CORS) is a form that was designed to be accessible to young people (Miller & Duncan, 2000 as cited in Miller et al., 2003). Clients rate themselves and report on how well they are doing personally, in relation to family and friends and at school, with an option to rate their overall sense of well-being. Each domain consists of a straight line, and the client can place a mark at any point on the ruler to indicate lower or higher levels of functioning for each area of their lives. Initially, this form was used as a conversation starter and to help develop therapeutic rapport with Flora. She scored herself a 6 (out of 10) in all domains, indicating difficulties regarding personal well-being, family relationships, and schoolwork.

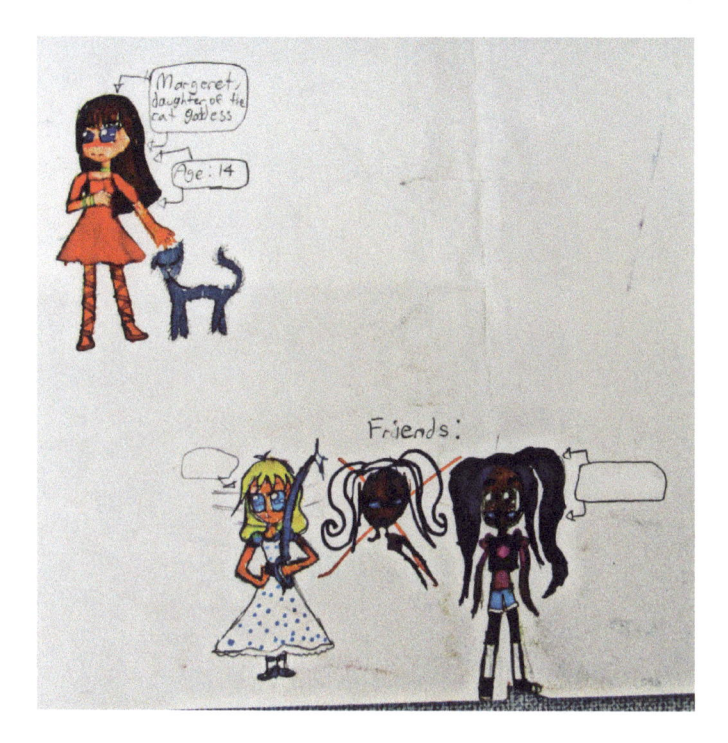

Figure 7.1 Friends

In relation to her art expression in these sessions, Flora would regularly draw cartoon characters and establish worlds for them to inhabit. However, she rarely provided a narrative for these characters and, generally, worked silently. While Flora seemed protective of her innermost thoughts and feelings, her characters (Figure 7.1) suggested that there was a rich inner world behind them.

Malchiodi (2020) states that psychological trauma can be a life-changing experience that affects multiple facets of health and wellbeing including memory, social engagement, and quality of life. Flora was dealing with multiple difficult life events at that time, including foster care and related attachment issues, separation from her family of origin, and beginning therapy pertaining to an indecent assault. The assault had led to heightened anxiety, mistrust, and confusion.

> Expressive arts therapies – the purposeful application of art, music, dance/movement, dramatic enactment, creative writing, and imaginative play – are largely nonverbal ways of self-expression of feelings and perceptions. More importantly, they are action-oriented and tap implicit, embodied experiences of trauma that can defy expression through verbal therapy or logic.
>
> (Malchiodi, 2020, p. 1)

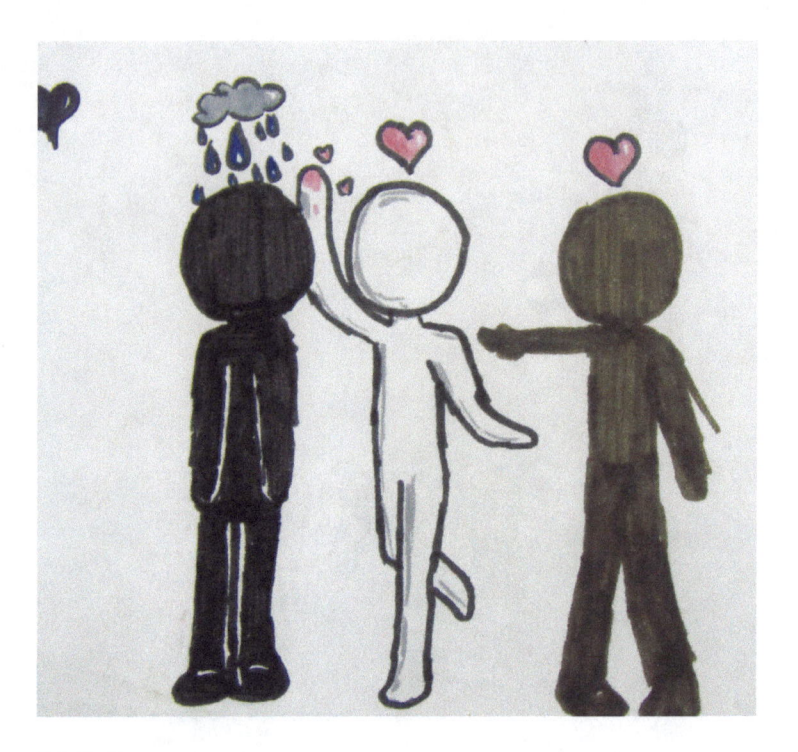

Figure 7.2 Feelings

In the assessment phase, Flora articulated that she wanted to work on being brave. There were aspects of the characters that she drew in her earlier sessions that seemed to bring to light qualities that Flora wanted to develop, such as confidence and pride in her achievements, and courage. Throughout her therapy, Flora's characters continued to express aspects of her life that, initially, could not be verbalised, signalling a parallel process that gave voice and meaning to her feelings and experiences.

As Flora grew more comfortable within the therapeutic relationship, she ventured into sand tray work and utilised symbols to depict home life and personal needs, such as those relating to developing identity as a teenager and finding her place within her extended family. Partway through the therapy Flora's caregiver reported that Flora was more confident and was making new friends more readily. During this phase of more connectivity, I experienced Flora's work in a way that allowed for exploration of the issues bringing into focus the challenges that she was facing in her life. Figure 7.2, Feelings, refers to a session during which Flora could identify her moods, enabling her to articulate feelings of sadness. This experience provided her with the means to track her feelings in the weeks that followed the session. There were also challenges associated with sibling and peer interactions that led to feelings of loneliness and

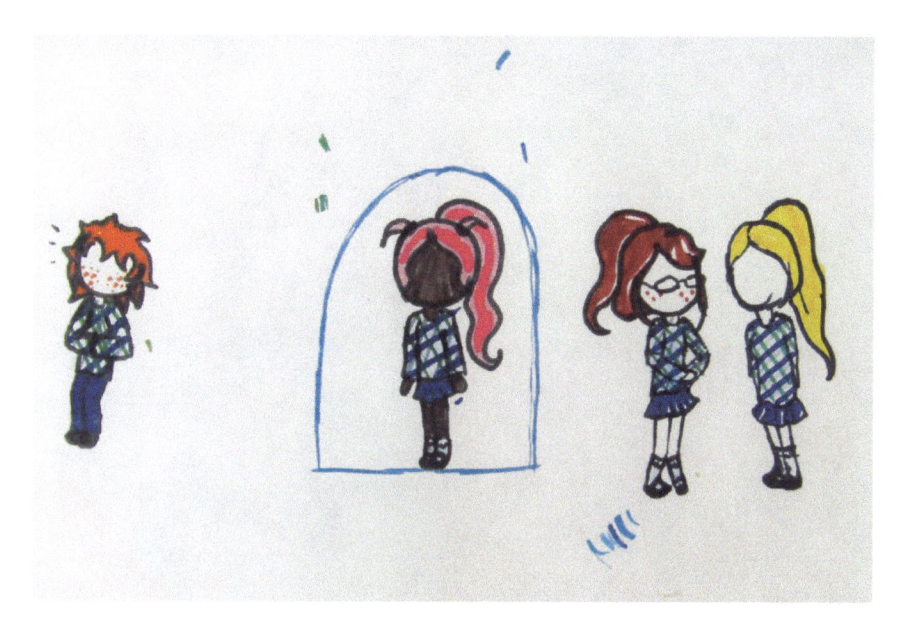

Figure 7.3 In a zone

isolation as reflected in Figure 7.3. In connection with Figure 7.3, In a Zone, Flora said that the girl in the blue enclosure was singled out and was 'in a zone'.

Once the therapeutic alliance is established and through empathic respond-ing, the client can grow in understanding of themselves and the world around them. This, in turn, can empower clients to make decisions regarding their lives. As the work intensified, and having explored her feelings about her fam-ily, our work together focused on peer relationships and Flora's need for wid-ening her social circle. Flora had begun to put words to her drawings and displayed more confidence in her interactions with me and with others. As the work progressed, Flora talked about the stories that she wrote alongside the drawings, bringing richness and a sense of deepening of her personal work.

In the following months, there were further changes and disruptions as Flora was transferred to another caregiver. This was a difficult transition for Flora; however, there was a promise of finding a home for life with her new family. A meeting with her new caregivers soon established a collaborative working relationship that supported Flora's stability and safety.

New versions of Flora's creations emerged as she expressed both internal and external changes. In the sessions that followed, a greater range of facial expressions and use of verbal language were observed. Visualisation and relaxa-tion exercises were introduced, and Flora responded positively to these as well. Malchiodi (2008) addresses the use of self-management techniques, including visualisation and art to help regulate intense emotions and as tools to support

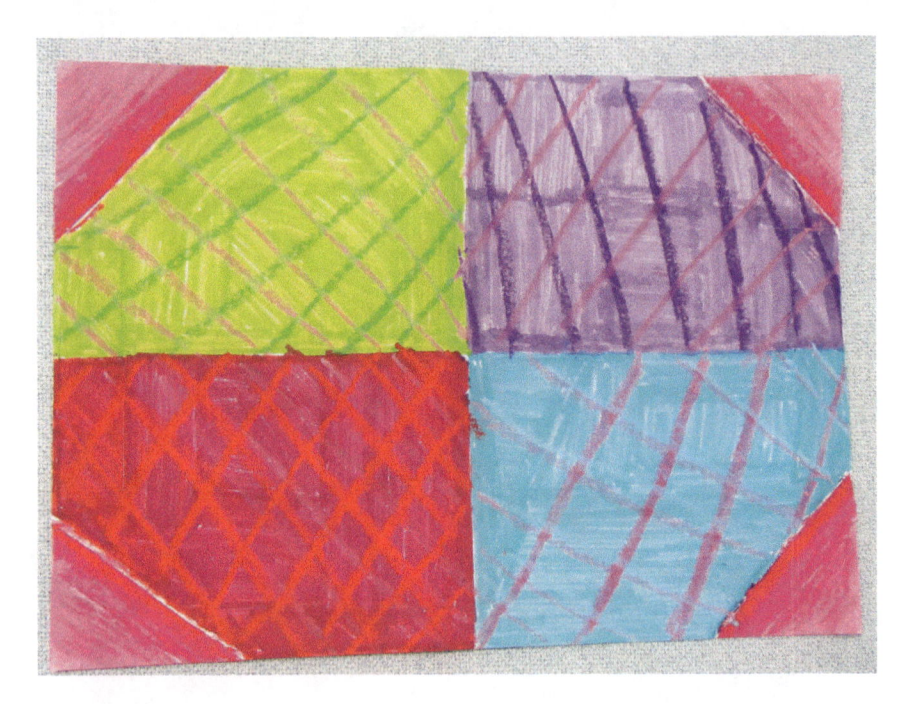

Figure 7.4 Diamond

grounding in trauma work. Murdock (1987) uses guided imagery with children and integrates learning, creativity, and relaxation. She suggests that children can learn more when they are relaxed. Murdock (1987) contends that "learning occurs throughout the entire brain" (p. 7). Pribram (1991) cited research indicating that memory is stored throughout the brain and concluded that exercises that enhance a client's ability to relax and use visual imagery would give them greater access to stored memories, bringing them into consciousness and facilitating processing and meaning-making.

At this stage in her therapy, Flora was becoming more communicative regarding her drawings and her characters depicted a more positive outlook on life. Flora enjoyed playing with colour and said that Figure 7.4 reminded her of a diamond. In sand play literature, minerals can symbolise stability, permanence, and strength. According to Boik and Goodwin (2000) "cut and shaped jewel-like stones can signify the soul shaped from the rough irregular stone into a beautiful treasure, the gem or the jewel" (p. 44). It is possible that Flora's depiction of a diamond in her artwork alluded to establishing a deeper connection with the centre of her essential self or soul, indicative of a shift in her self-perception. Flora was also able to articulate aspects of the story that accompanied Figure 7.5 and said that Margaret was the daughter of the cat goddess. She had set off on an adventure. Flora explained that the girl was growing up and the cat was Margaret's guide.

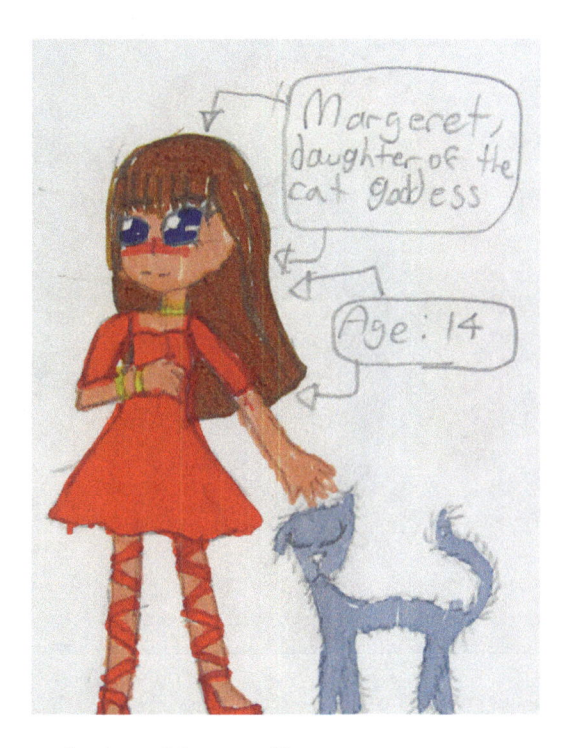

Figure 7.5 Margaret, daughter of the cat goddess

The thread running through Flora's therapy and her imagery signalled an expansion of the use of imaginative capacities. Imagination and creative expression are fundamental principles in the arts therapies and as such, developing imagination is often one of the primary goals of therapy. McNiff (2004) declares that "life is an ongoing practice of sensitivity and cooperation in which imagination and the physical world influence one another" (p. 85). According to McNiff (2004), clinical treatment involves "an empathic and imaginal engagement of the problem as a generative force, and not just a sign that something is wrong" (p. 85). Imagination provides a portal to a new way of being in the world, facilitating the flow of ideas and enabling our clients to develop greater problem-solving capacities. McNiff (2004) explains that clients can "experience depth and meaning by staying with the characters of imagination, letting them speak, reveal themselves and emerge according to their respective natures" (p. 86). McNiff has written extensively about the role of imagination and creativity in the healing process and suggested that therapy becomes a creative collaboration with imagination and the world from which it emanates. He declared that "the process generally requires us to relax the self so that imagination can treat itself within the context of its innate wisdom" (McNiff, 2004, p. 88).

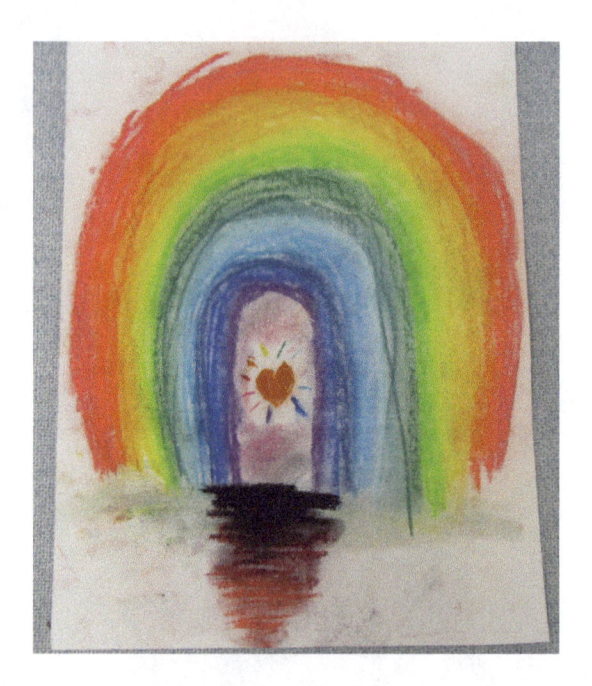

Figure 7.6 Life is about creating myself

Creative expression in its many forms can deepen the connection with one's true self and can facilitate a process of change and transformation. According to Csikszentmihaly (1996) creativity results from the interaction between a person's thoughts and a sociocultural context. He speaks about an inner conviction and a sense of confidence that arises when a person involved in creative expression experiences this as valuable. Creativity enables the individual "to bring into existence something genuinely new that is valued enough to be added to the culture" (Csikszentmihaly, 1996, p. 25). There was a subtle yet profound change in Flora especially in the latter stages of therapy and this was evidenced in her final drawings. Flora was able to give expression to her inner world through her creations in an atmosphere of acceptance and care. She had also become more confident; there was a reduction in anxiety symptoms associated with the traumatic incident and she was settled in her environment. This enabled Flora to develop her sense of self, by connecting with her own thoughts and feelings.

In the last few sessions of art therapy, Flora seemed more expressive and more open to the world. On one occasion, she took an interest in a picture on the wall in the clinic rooms. The picture was accompanied by these words: "Life isn't about finding yourself; life is about creating yourself". Flora, unprompted, used these words as inspiration and created her next picture. In that session, Flora created a drawing of a rainbow (Figure 7.6) and expressed her associated thoughts in one sentence 'my soul matters'. For the remainder of the session, we explored together her innermost aspirations.

Flora used the term *soul* for the first time near the completion of therapy. Kalsched (2013) speaks about soul as a "vital animating core of our embodied selves – a certain essential something that links us to each other, to the divine and to the exquisite beauties of the natural and cultural worlds" (p. 10). Jung addressed the question of soul and the experience of the spiritual, alluding to this realm with an attitude that inspires awe and worship of something beyond the ego. According to Kalsched (2013), early relational trauma results from the fact that we are often given more to experience in life than we can bear to experience consciously. It is possible that Flora lost sight of aspects of herself that were then able to resurface and find renewed expression and vitality through art therapy.

In *Art as Medicine*, McNiff (1992) advocates for a therapy of the imagination and describes his pioneering methods of art therapy including interpretation through storytelling, creative collaboration, and dialoguing with images. McNiff also refers to the soul and suggests that the term refers to a person's essential nature. In the introduction to his book, McNiff speaks of soul as an inner movement or stirring, the force of creative animation and vitality. He alludes to a therapeutic process through creative engagement that allows the individual to experience themselves more deeply (McNiff, 1992). McNiff's approach to art psychotherapy is to follow the phases from creation to reflection, signalling that the medicinal agent is art itself. It was in this context that I witnessed and honoured Flora's art expressions, knowing and trusting the process of being present to the wisdom inherent in both the client and the process.

Discussion

The expressive therapies have emphasised the contribution made by neuroscience and neurobiology in support of the effectiveness of arts-based methods in the treatment of trauma, particularly with children and young people (Malchiodi, 2020). This body of work continues to provide the arts therapies with new ways to measure and identify what works and why it works. In addition, there is an emergence of a brain–body framework within the context of trauma-informed practice (Malchiodi, 2020). As such, the arts therapies represent a whole-brain approach as arts-based methods activate many parts of the brain. For example, art processes such as drawing and clay sculpting generate specific brain waves that simulate a meditative state and can reduce anxiety symptoms (Kruk et al., 2014).

Earlier in this chapter, I referred to two models that informed my work with Flora. The first of these is a relational framework (ATR–N) that draws on neuroscience (Figure 7.7), the dynamic interplay of brain and bodily systems and

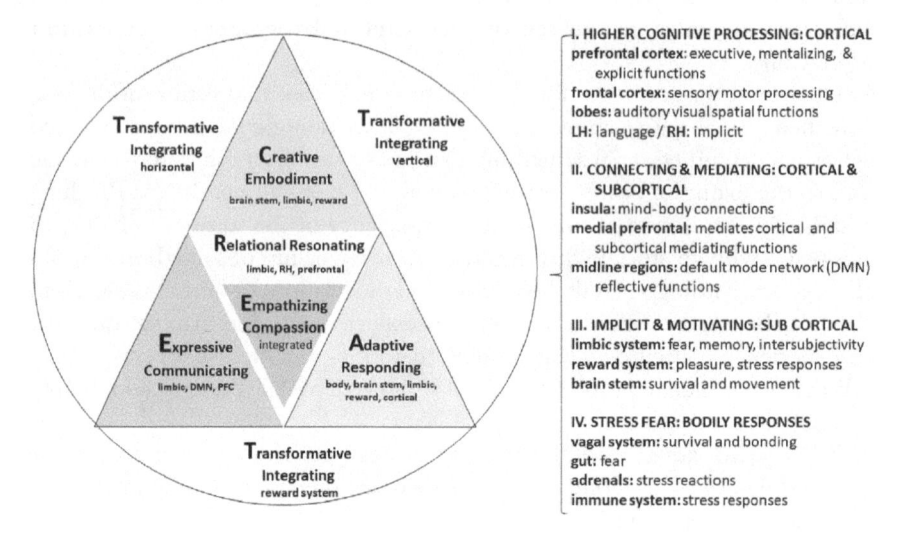

Figure 7.7 The dynamic interplay of brain and bodily systems and art therapy relational neuroscience principles

art therapy relational neuroscience principles (Hass-Cohen, adapted diagram, personal communication, 2021).

> The circular diagram indicates the main structures that each CREATE principle, Creative Embodiment, Relational Resonance, Expressive Communicating, Adaptive Responding, Transformative Integrating, Empathizing & Compassion is associated with. The chart on the right indicates four main interpersonal neurobiology pathways activated in CREATE. Transformative horizontal integration refers to right to left hemispheric connections, vertical integration includes bi-directional cortical-subcortical-bodily connections.
>
> (Permission Noah Hass-Cohen, personal communication, April 16, 2021)

A brief description of the six CREATE principles follows.

According to Hass-Cohen and Findlay (2015), the CREATE framework "underscores the neurological underpinnings of art therapy interventions and change, assisting art therapists in fine-tuning their clinical work and teaching practices" (p. 10). *Creative Embodiment* relates to the potential therapeutic effects of kinaesthetic artmaking and the rhythmic movement involved in artmaking. *Relational Resonating* refers to the positive effects of interpersonal interactions in the context of the therapeutic relationship with clients, which have the corresponding effect of promoting emotional regulation and contribute to attachment. Hass-Cohen refers to examples of Relational Resonating including offering and sharing media and working together. Such experiences can contribute towards establishing or re-establishing secure attachments. *Expressive Communicating* relates to stimulating emotional engagement within the art therapy environment. Hass-Cohen and Findlay (2015) propose that "this activation is likely to charge clients' neurological reward circuitry while helping to maintain a dynamic balance between excitation, pleasure and tranquillity" (p. 11). *Adaptive Responding* relates to the art therapist's capacity to provide an environment in which the client feels a degree of personal control, acceptance, resilience, and safety. This approach involves "simultaneous art making, meaning making, and contextual memory processing" (Hass-Cohen & Findlay, 2015, p. 11). This is particularly helpful for trauma clients as artmaking in this context can support re-framing of the trauma experience and generate solutions. Adaptive Responding leads to the fifth principle involving *Transformative Integrating*. At this level, clients can experience greater integration of the interpersonal self. "Under therapeutic conditions, symbol-making and verbalisation of art making can re-organise and re-structure implicit emotional memories" (Hass-Cohen & Findlay, 2015, p. 12). The sixth principle, *Empathising and Compassion*, relates to the development of insight and compassion toward oneself, toward others, and toward the art product. These principles demonstrate an interconnectedness that suggests a holistic approach to treatment, one that encompasses the creative process and its inherent value in promoting self-awareness and the role of imagination in problem-solving, and attends to emotional and cognitive functioning (Hass-Cohen & Findlay, 2015).

These CREATE principles found expression in my interactions with Flora during her art therapy process. The principle of Relational Resonating is evident in a conscious intention to provide Flora with a choice of art materials from the beginning of her therapy to encourage self-mastery, which also reflects an important aspect of trauma work. Flora's enthusiasm for artmaking and investment in the process supported by my verbal and non-verbal responses facilitated Flora's engagement with meaning-making over time and created space for fuller emotional expression. The principle of Expressive Communicating is addressed in this work in terms of stimulating motivation and emotional expression while Relational Resonating addresses the importance of the therapeutic relationship that can support and promote psychobiological changes. The principle of Adaptive Responding is seen in my attempts to "desensitise emotions and memories and generate solutions" (Hass-Cohen & Findlay, 2015, p. 11). This relates to a time when Flora was feeling more comfortable in her therapy, and we worked with relaxation and visualisation to facilitate the processing of traumatic memories. This principle was also reflected in Flora's ability to speak about some of her challenges in dealing with family relationships. The sixth principle of Empathising and Compassion refers to the latter stages of Flora's art therapy, a time that saw a deepening of our work together, when we explored, compassionately, Flora's deeper needs in relation to her emerging sense of self. This aspect was reflected in her work and in verbalisation that her soul matters as depicted in Figure 7.6. At this point in her therapy Flora had acquired increased adaptability and a newfound sense of well-being. In this context, creativity and imagination gained greater expression and supported resiliency.

Fonagy and Allison (2014) have written about mentalisation based treatment and suggest that mentalising is a key aspect of the therapeutic process. They state that "the experience of feeling thought about in therapy makes us feel safe enough to think about ourselves in relation to our world, and to learn something new about that world and how we operate in it" (Fonagy & Allison, 2014, p. 375). Hass–Cohen and Findlay (2015) state that "the study of mentalising suggests that successful social mentalising is tied to secure attachment, which is key to coherent intersubjectivity and therefore to successfully partaking in learning and social contexts" (p. 73).

Hass–Cohen and Findlay (2015) have paid particular attention in their research to the connections between neuroscience and interpersonal neurobiology in an attempt to gain a better understanding of brain activity, attachment theories, and art therapy as an approach to treatment. King (2016) in her review of Hass–Cohen and Findlay's work signalled that the CREATE principles address internal working models through the use of art materials. King (2016) suggested that "the flexibility of the brain contributes to internal working models of the mind and influences attachment patterns throughout the course of therapy" (p. 51). This is an important consideration in the context of the therapeutic alliance as a healing agent as well.

Attachment is a core feature of resilience and part of our work as clinicians involves helping clients build resilience. Maston (2001) states that "resilience does not come from rare and special abilities, but from the everyday magic of ordinary, normative human resources in the minds, brains, and bodies of children, in their families, and in their communities" (p. 235).

Neuroscience has contributed to clarifying what happens when individuals make art and studies of the mirror neuron system (Gallese, 2003: Gallese et al., 2004) have brought together neuroscience research, theories of attachment, art, and empathy. Arnheim (1966, as cited in Franklin, 2010, p. 163) considered expression and perception as intimately related: "This view considers affect to exist in the actual object of perception" (p. 163). Empathy can help locate emotional content in visual imagery. Book (1988) addresses empathy by suggesting that it indicates attuned understanding, which gives access to a client's internal world. Franklin (2010) suggests that therapists, through empathic attunement, can help clients feel seen and develop empathy for themselves and others. These findings strengthen the value of employing art therapy with clients who are non-verbal or who struggle to communicate emotions and articulate cognitions related to traumatic experiences.

Beres (2012) defines imagination as "the action of imagining or forming a mental concept of what is not actually present to the senses" and "as the result of this, a mental image or idea" (p. 252). Beres (2012) also contends that the products of imagination consist of the fantasy, the thought, the dream, and the symbol (p. 252). Flora was offered artmaking as a way of reaching within to explore her deepest emotions, thoughts, fears, and motivations. Over time, the use of this creative language and encouragement towards self-expression afforded Flora new insights and renewed confidence.

A second model was used to review my work with Flora in the context of stages of therapy (de Rivera, 1992). de Rivera refers to the psychotherapeutic relationship in four stages: commitment, process, change and termination. The material presented in this chapter refers to the latter stages of process and change as these provided the most observable information in relation to Flora's presentation, engagement in therapy and insight-oriented work. de Rivera (1992, p. 2) refers to the stages of *process* and *change* as significant in terms of acquiring new information relating to the client and ensuring the consolidation of therapeutic gains. The understanding of stages of therapy can assist clinicians to provide a carefully titrated approach to treatment. This was helpful in Flora's case as her engagement was initially tentative and there was a risk that she might disengage from therapy at any time.

Specifically, de Rivera identifies the process as a stage that involves searching for patterns and new information, as well as working towards consolidation. This is considered to be the most complex stage and incorporates the sensation of psychic movement (de Rivera, 1992, p. 3). de Rivera explains that during this phase the client may experience that they are becoming aware of something. de Rivera proposes that this is more important than what the client is becoming aware of. This author also refers to vicious circles in relation to patterns that are maladaptive and the necessity to bring these patterns into awareness and to work collaboratively with clients to break the cycle. During our time together, I had a felt sense that Flora might readily revert to a pattern of withdrawal and dissociation due to her history of trauma, even after she began to put words to her images and engaged in more expressive work. It was therefore important to endeavour to be more attuned to the subtle nuances in our relationship in order to support her progress in therapy. The stage of therapy defined as change comprises sub-phases that have been referred to as relinquish, initiate, and sustain (de Rivera, 1992). This stage alludes to new beginnings; the experience of a new, healthier psychic life; and developing a level of resilience and skills to assist the client to protect and maintain the newly acquired strengths. This was evidenced in the later stages of Flora's therapy when she found her voice and was able to articulate her deeper needs, both in therapy and at home. This was also a time when there were observable differences in levels of self-confidence and assertiveness.

The field of therapeutic change process research advocates for the importance of studying the linguistic products of change (e.g. activities, tasks, journaling) in order to better understand therapeutic change as it relates to process and outcomes (Kazdin & Nock, 2003; Imel et al., 2015 as cited in Smink et al., 2019). In considering health-related outcomes for our clients and finding appropriate research methodology, there is an argument for tracking the process of change in all its manifestations to raise our awareness as clinicians and to enhance our ethical practice.

I suggest that there are parallels between these two models (ATR-N and de Rivera's process of change) that serve to corroborate Flora's art therapy experiences as presented in this chapter.

Conclusion

Over a period of several months of art therapy, Flora's images told a story of a developing sense of self, cultural identification, and attachment difficulties in the context of her history of trauma. Art therapy provided a setting for Flora's nonverbal explorations, and the neuroscience of imagination supported meaning-making and the work of making the unconscious conscious. The work with Flora and her art expressions were reviewed in this chapter in the context of two models that addressed, respectively, the importance of relational neuroscience in the context of art therapy supported by an understanding of theories of change that can help strengthen the validity of outcomes in the arts therapies.

When working with children and young persons, it is important to consider the impact of environmental and familial influences. During our time together, Flora moved to a home for life, and the stability of her environment with caring foster parents would have been a factor in her recovery. Art therapy appeared to serve Flora's needs for self-expression and helped mobilise and awaken functions that led to changes in behaviour while supporting her emotional and cognitive development.

At the beginning of our work together, Flora scored herself a 6 in all domains of the CORS scale (personal, familial, and social). Towards the end of her therapy, Flora scored herself a 9 in each of these domains, indicating improvements in her overall sense of well-being. This outcome was supported by Flora's own verbal feedback and presentation.

Three years after the art therapy intervention, I was able to meet with Flora for a follow-up session. She was 16 years old at the time and was settled in her home and school life. When I enquired about what had changed, Flora said that she was feeling much more confident and was making plans for her future. She was talkative, smiled with ease and presented as more self-assured. Even though we met following disruptions to her school life caused by COVID-19 restrictions, Flora was optimistic about the future and glad to return to school, signalling her resiliency and capacity to self-manage.

According to Malchiodi (2020),

> addressing trauma in children and adults is not a one-size-fits-all endeavour. Effective intervention includes viewing individuals not only through the acute or chronic events they have experienced, but also through the interpersonal, cultural, social and ecological factors that form the context for their perceptions and trauma-related reactions.
>
> (p. 36)

The expressive arts therapies have a role in trauma-informed work as they provide a holistic approach to treatment encompassing emotional, cognitive, physical, and spiritual considerations. The arts therapies offer a window into the self and can assist with the integration of all the senses and support recovery. McNiff (2009) summarised this by saying that "when art and psychotherapy are joined, the scope and depth of each can be expanded, and when working together, they are tied to the continuities of humanity's history of healing" (p. 259).

Acknowledgements

I wish to express my sincere thanks to Caroline Miller for our collaboration and for the immense opportunity to learn and grow throughout this project. Thank you to Flora, who inspired me to share her story and creative journey; to Auckland University of Technology for the support I received and encouragement to undertake research; to Noah Hass-Cohen and colleagues for their work in bringing the arts therapies into the age of neuroscience and interpersonal neurobiology; and to our colleagues and fellow writers with whom we share this book. Their work serves to strengthen the arts therapies community around the world and affirm the value of the arts in healing.

References

Beres, D. (2012, April 8). The psychoanalytic psychology of imagination. *Journal of the American Psychoanalytic Association, 1960,* 252–269. https://doi.org/10.1177/000306516000800202

Boik, B. L., & Goodwin, E. A. (2000). *Sandplay therapy a step-by-step manual for psychotherapists of diverse orientations.* W. W. Norton.

Book, H. E. (1988). Empathy: Misconceptions and misuses in psychotherapy. *American Journal of Psychiatry, 145,* 420–424.

British Association of Art Therapists. (2020, February 7). *International art therapy practice research inaugural conference report – day three: 13th July 2019.* www.baat.org/About-BAAT/Blog/252/International-Art-Therapy-Practice-Research-Inaugural-Conference-report-Day-Three-13th-July-2019.

Chodorow, J. (2006). Active imagination. In R. K. Papadopoulos (Ed.), *The handbook of Jungian psychology: Theory, practice and applications* (pp. 215–243). Taylor & Francis Group.

Csikszentmihalyi, M. (1996). *Creativity flow and the psychology of discovery and invention.* Harper Collins.

de Rivera, J. L. G. (1992). The stages of psychotherapy. *European Journal of Psychiatry, 6*(1), 51–58.

Fonagy, P., & Allison, E. (2014). The role of mentalising and epistemic trust in the therapeutic relationship. *Psychotherapy, 51*(3), 372–380.

Franklin, M. (2010). Affect regulation, mirror neurons, and the third hand: Formulating mindful empathic art interventions. *Journal of the American Art therapy Association, 27*(4), 160–167. doi:10.1080/07421656.2010.10129385

Gallese, V. (2003). The roots of empathy: The shared manifold hypothesis and the neural basis of intersubjectivity. *Psychopathology, 36,* 171–180.

Gallese, V., Keysers, C., & Rizzolati, G. (2004). A unifying view of social cognition. *Trends in Cognitive Science, 8,* 396–403.

Hass-Cohen, N., & Findlay, J. C. (2015). *Art therapy and the neuroscience of relationships, creativity and resiliency skills and practices.* W. W. Norton.

Hogan, S. (2015). *Art therapy theories, a critical introduction.* Routledge.

Kalsched, D. (2013). *Trauma and the soul, a psycho-spiritual approach to human development and its interruption.* Routledge.

Kapitan, L. (Ed.). (2010). The empathic imagination of art therapy: Good for the brain? *Art Therapy Journal of the American Art Therapy Association, 27*(4), 158–159. https://doi.org/1 0.1080/07421656.2010.10129384

Kazdin, A. E., & Nock, M. K. (2003). Delineating mechanisms of change in child and adolescent therapy: Methodological issues and research recommendations. *Journal of* Child Psychology and Psychiatry, 44(8), 1116–1129.

King, J. L. (2016). Art therapy and the neuroscience of relationships, creativity and resiliency: Skills and practices. *Journal of the American Art Therapy Association, 33*(1), pp. 51–53.

Klorer, P. G. (2017). The neuroscience of art therapy and trauma. In *Expressive therapy with traumatized children* (pp. 9–16). Rowman & Littlefield.

Kruk, K. A., Aravich, P. F., Deaver, S. P., & de Beus, R. (2014). Comparison of brain activity during drawing and clay sculpting: A preliminary qEEG study. *Art Therapy: Journal of the American Art Therapy Association, 31*(2), 52–60.

Malchiodi, C. A. (2008). *Creative interventions with traumatised children.* Guilford Press.

Malchiodi, C. A. (2020). *Trauma and expressive arts therapy, brain, body and imagination in the healing process.* Guilford Press.

Maston, A. S. (2001). Ordinary magic: Resilience processes in development. *American Psychologist, 56*(3), 227–238.

McNamee, C. M. (2003). Bilateral art: Facilitating systemic integration and balance. *The Arts in Psychotherapy, 30,* 283–292.

McNamee, C. M. (2006). Experiences in bilateral art: A retrospective study. *Art Therapy: Journal of the American Art Therapy Association, 23*(1), 7–13. https://doi.101.1080/074216 56.2006.10129526

McNiff, S. (1992). *Art as medicine, creating a therapy of the imagination.* Shambhala Publications.

McNiff, S. (2004). *Art heals, how creativity cures the soul.* Shambhala Publications.

McNiff, S. (2009). *Integrating the arts in therapy: History, theory, and practice.* Charles C. Thomas.

Miller, C. (Ed.). (2014). *Assessment and outcomes in the arts therapies: A person-centred approach.* Jessica Kingsley.

Miller, S. D., Duncan, B. L., Brown, J., Sparks, J. A., & Claud, D. A. (2003). The outcome rating scale: A preliminary study of the reliability, validity and feasibility of a brief visual analog measure. *Journal of Brief Therapy, 2*(2), 91–100.

Moon, C. H. (2002). *Studio art therapy, cultivating the artist identity in the art therapist.* Jessica Kingsley.

Murdock, M. (1987). *Spinning inward using guided imagery with children for learning, creativity and relaxation.* Shambhala.

Papadopoulos, R. K. (2006). *The handbook of Jungian psychology: Theory, practice and applications* (pp. 215–243). Taylor & Francis Group.

Pribram, K. H. (1991). *Brain and perception: Holonomy and structure in figural processing.* Psychology Press.

Rubin, J. A. (1999). *Art therapy, an introduction.* Taylor & Francis.

Rubin, J. A. (2001). *Approaches to art therapy, theory & technique.* Brunner-Routledge.

Smink, W. A. C., Fox, J.-P., Tjong Kim Sang, E., Sools, A. M., Westerhof, G. J., & Veld-kamp, B. P. (2019). Understanding therapeutic change process research through multilevel modelling and text mining. *Frontiers in Psychology, 10*(1186). https://doi.org/10.3389/fpsyg.2019.01186

Stevens, A. (1982). *Archetype, a natural history of the self.* Routledge.

Additional reading

Crenshaw, D. A., Brooks, R., & Goldstein, S. (2015). *Play therapy interventions to enhance resilience.* Guilford Press.

Heidegger, M. (1953). *Introduction to metaphysics.* Yale University Press.

Holmqvist, G., Roxberg, A., Larsson, I., & Lundqvist-Persson, C. (2017). What art thera-pists consider to be patient's inner change and how it may appear during art therapy. *The Arts in Psychotherapy, 56,* 45–52. https://doi.org/10.1016/j.aip.2017.07.005

King, J. L. (Ed.). (2016). *Art therapy, trauma and neuroscience, theoretical and practical perspectives.* Routledge.

Weber, K. (2019). *The study of neurological response in art therapy and trauma: A literature review.* Lesley University. https://digitalcommons.lesley.edu/cgi/viewcontent.cgi?article=1136 &context=expressive_theses.

8 Singing all together in the CeleBRation Choir

A music therapist's perspective on community singing for adults who have neurogenic communication difficulties

Alison Talmage

Prelude: just sing!

Singing has been a constant in my life as a musician, teacher, and music therapist. My childhood and adolescence were enriched through choirs and songwriting. As a primary school teacher, I facilitated classroom singing, choir performances, and school shows. Music therapy training opened a world of playful vocal improvisation with non-verbal children. My repertoire broadened through the preferred songs and cultural identities of clients aged a few months to 100.

Today, community choirs are flourishing in communities across the world. Research evidence supports the salutogenic benefits of singing. Specialist choirs for people with specific health needs have been established by music therapists, community musicians, speech-language therapists, and others. Yet even now I meet too many people wounded by, at best, careless or, at worst, cruel words from teachers, conductors, or peers, creating a phenomenon of *selective mutism for singing* (West, 2009). One music therapy participant turned to poetry to express personal experiences and feelings as a non-singer and the irony of hearing that singing might ameliorate the voice symptoms of Parkinson's disease (Hicks, 2018).

In this chapter, I discuss therapeutic singing, with illustrations from my work with the CeleBRation Choir, whose members have neurogenic communication difficulties – problems resulting from a neurological condition. In the choir, singing is acknowledged as a multifaceted, social activity reflecting our personal and shared values. The intrinsic aesthetic pleasure and social functions of group singing provide a framework for the second, instrumental purpose of maintaining, maximising, or recovering communication abilities. Our repertoire includes specially composed songs, as well as participants' own favourite music. Throughout this chapter I have prefaced sections with song lyrics – most are from a song that gave the choir a voice in disseminating findings of the SPICCATO Study (Stroke and Parkinson's: Investigating Community Choirs and Therapeutic Outcomes; Fogg-Rogers et al., 2016; Talmage et al., 2013).

DOI: 10.4324/9781003082897-12

The CeleBRation Choir

> Monday afternoons at university,
> The CBR is the place to be,
> Choral singing is our therapy,
> Oh, we all love the CeleBRation Choir!
> *(Talmage et al., 2013, p. 47)*

The CeleBRation Choir is a music therapist-led group for adults who have neurogenic communication difficulties – problems with voice, speech, language, or memory, resulting from a neurological condition such as stroke, Parkinson's disease, dementia, or traumatic brain injury. *CeleBRation* highlights our affiliation with the University of Auckland's Centre for Brain Research (CBR), as well as participants' determination to make the most of life. Established in 2009, CeleBRation Choir was New Zealand's first *neurological choir*, an approach that crosses diagnostic boundaries. Community choirs have an inclusive ethos but attract predominantly well or non-disabled singers. Narrow, diagnostic criteria underpin aphasia choirs, Parkinson's choirs, memory choirs, and other treatment programmes. In contrast, while guided by the CBR's purpose, the CeleBRation Choir brings together people living with varied neurological conditions, supportive partners, family members, carers, and volunteers. Other neurological choirs in New Zealand have followed this model (Music Therapy New Zealand, 2019). Furthermore, in an era that values service users' voices, CeleBRation Choir members were the first music therapy participants to attend a New Zealand music therapy conference (Rickson, 2012).

In many ways neurological choirs resemble regular community choirs – groups of people warming up, making music together, and enjoying a varied repertoire of songs of manageable complexity. The difference lies in the choice of exercises, methods of song leading and arranging, and an emphasis on presence, camaraderie, enjoyment, effort, and improvement, rather than musical perfection. Our sense of community is reflected in our repertoire, such as the round, "Singing All Together" (Figure 8.1).

In our music-centred choir programme, individual communication difficulties are considered from a holistic biopsychosocial-spiritual perspective (Hatala, 2013). In our context of Aotearoa New Zealand, a holistic indigenous model, *Te Whare Tapa Whā*, is relevant, particularly for our New Zealand Māori participants, focusing on spiritual, mental, physical, and family health (Durie, 1985; Purdy, 2020). Daveson's (2008) Meta-Model of Music Therapy in Neuro-Disability (MIND) also offers a person-centred framework of "restorative, compensatory and psycho-social-emotional approaches" (p. 70). In the choir, the MIND approach underpins opportunities for participants to focus on the recovery of communication skills or to experience a new activity, as well as prioritising well-being. Whereas a treatment approach typically leads to separate interventions for people with specific diagnoses, our programme

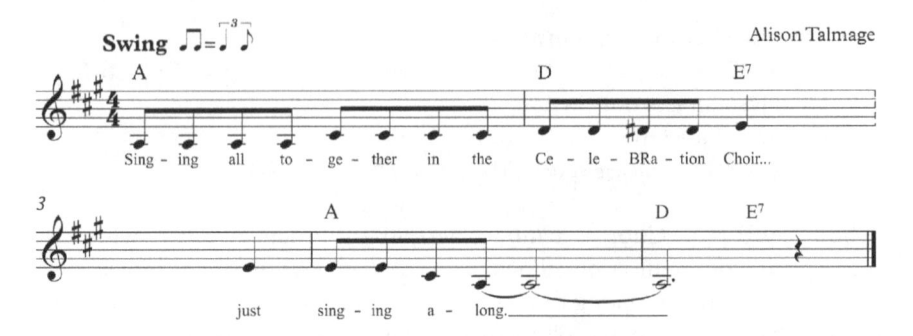

Figure 8.1 "Singing All Together" (extract; Talmage, 2020d) Note: Dotted lines indicate where bars of a song are omitted.

simultaneously targets a range of communication skills, explores alternative ways of participating, and nurtures a sense of belonging and enjoyment.

Moving beyond our participants' enthusiasm for the choir, what is the neuroscientific basis for this approach? Why encourage someone with a communication difficulty to sing? What are the therapeutic outcomes?

Singing and quality of life

> Quality of life is better if you sing,
> Surrounded by friends and all the love they bring,
> Singing cheers you up, it's a positive thing,
> Oh, we all love the CeleBRation Choir!
> *(Talmage et al., 2013, p. 48)*

Many international studies have reported a positive correlation between community singing and well-being for the general population and encouraging findings for singing interventions for people with a range of specific health issues. This resonates with our research that has found higher than expected self-reported quality of life for participants in neurological choirs (Jenkins et al., 2017).

The CeleBRation Choir values *choral singing therapy* for people with communication difficulties (Fogg-Rogers et al., 2016; Talmage et al., 2013). Old and new members alike are made welcome in weekly, semi-open sessions. The greatest surprise for me has been the collective enthusiasm for public performance at university functions, in rest homes, and in the wider community. An intergenerational performance with a local school led to a reciprocal invitation to participate in the primary schools' music festival in the town hall. The choir has twice performed in the cathedral – once in a combined choirs' concert and once to support Distinguished Professor Sir Richard Faull, founder of the CBR (Radio New Zealand, 2013). A television appearance promoted New Zealand's inaugural Music Therapy Week (TVNZ, 2016), and a short documentary film about the choir, named after Roger Hicks's poem, was selected for the 2020 New Zealand Documentary Edge Film Festival (Chadha, 2019). Many members forego anonymity to share their experiences openly with the wider community (CeleBRation Choir, 2020; Christian, 2016; Johnston, 2019; White, 2018).

The joy, camaraderie, and therapeutic benefits of singing are experiences that the choir members value and advocate for others like themselves. Their active support for research is motivated by curiosity about how singing works, opportunities to contribute to new knowledge formation, and the hope of more choirs for more people like themselves.

Neurogenic communication difficulties

Brain injury or disease can affect functioning in many domains – physical, sensory, cognitive, psychosocial, and communication. *Neurogenic* conditions are caused by changes in the brain or nervous system, in contrast to *psychogenic* symptoms caused by psychological factors. While the challenges depend on the individual's specific diagnosis and life circumstances, many people experience a reduced quality of life marked by loss of professional, leisure and social activities. Music-based approaches within neurorehabilitation are valuable because music perception and music-making recruit networks across the whole brain (Koelsch, 2012). The CeleBRation Choir focus on communication particularly supports people living with aphasia, Parkinson's disease, or dementia.

Aphasia

> Group data show, by a stroke of luck,
> You can sing in the choir and you won't feel stuck,
> Your words will feel simpler to construct,
> Oh, we all love the CeleBRation Choir!
> *(Talmage et al., 2013, p. 47)*

Aphasia is a chronic impairment of expressive and/or receptive language that also affects reading and writing (Brady et al., 2016). Of the many types of aphasia, post-stroke non-fluent (or Broca's) aphasia is most common among our choir members. Stroke predominantly, but not exclusively, affects older people. With an annual incidence of 12 million strokes globally, stroke is the second-most common cause of death worldwide (after heart disease) for people aged 50 and older and a significant cause of disability (GBD 2019 Diseases and Injuries Collaborators, 2020). About 85% of strokes are *ischaemic* (caused by a blockage, usually a blood clot) and 15% *haemorrhagic* (caused by bleeding in an artery in the brain; Ward & Cannon, 2018). Approximately one third of stroke survivors have aphasia – and effective speech-language therapy treatment and social programmes unfortunately have high attrition rates (Brady et al., 2016). Australian researchers have recommended a person-centred approach in which the individual's priorities would guide participation in psychosocial and/or language programmes (Worrall et al., 2017) – this echoes Daveson's (2008) approach discussed earlier.

Support for singing-based aphasia rehabilitation is premised on the overlapping neural networks for speech and singing. It is well known that stroke survivors who have non-fluent aphasia (characterised by hesitant, telegraphic speech with reduced prosody) often retain the ability to sing, and many aphasia choirs have been established around the world. Neuroimaging studies show the involvement of temporal, frontal, and parietal lobes in processing both language and music, although there are specialist pathways within these regions (Särkämö & Sihvonen, 2018). Research findings are encouraging, but studies to date have been small scale. Participants in an Australian aphasia choir reported improvements in confidence, peer support, mood, motivation, and communication (Tamplin et al., 2013). Similarly, participants with aphasia in a neurological choir perceived singing as beneficial in managing social isolation, low mood, and communication difficulties (Fogg-Rogers et al., 2016).

In successful singing-based therapy for aphasia rehabilitation, there is debate as to the relative importance of rhythm and pitch (Stahl et al., 2011; Zumbansen et al., 2014). A small-scale study demonstrated that a rhythm-based singing approach was acceptable to CeleBRation Choir participants and proposed a further comparison of rhythmic and melody-based approaches (Thompson et al., 2017). Whether one element or the other eventually proves more important, our participants value a collaborative, music-centred focus.

Parkinson's disease

> Your voice will be louder, tuneful and strong,
> When you've lots to say, your breath will be long,
> You know you've a voice, and you are not wrong,
> Oh, we all love the CeleBRation Choir!
> *(Talmage et al., 2013, p. 47)*

Parkinson's disease is a progressive neurological disorder associated with reduced dopamine production by the substantia nigra in the midbrain and causing a range of motor and non-motor symptoms (Martinez-Martin et al., 2015). Worldwide, 10 million people live with Parkinson's. About 89% have *hypokinetic dysarthria*, a cluster of voice and speech problems. Dysarthria affects all aspects of speech production – respiration, voice quality, resonance, articulation, and prosody. No consistent speech improvement has been found through the usual medical treatments for Parkinson's – L-dopa medication and deep-brain stimulation surgery (Dashtipour et al., 2018).

Physiological problems that might cause hypokinetic dysarthria include cueing, planning, and initiating articulatory movements; scaling and effort in laryngeal movements; sensory processing and perception of speech volume; timing and rhythmicity; emotional expression; and conscious or unconscious self-monitoring (Sapir, 2014). Assessment relies on a combination of perceptual, acoustic, and video endoscopy assessments and self-reports. Speech-language therapy, particularly the Lee Silverman Voice Treatment, is the usual treatment approach, targeting loudness, speech rate and clarity through breathing, phonation (voicing), articulation, and self-monitoring techniques.

Singing has been proposed as an alternative approach (Di Benedetto et al., 2009). The SPICCATO study demonstrated the practicality and acceptability of a choir approach and mixed-methods research, illustrated through a published case study (Talmage et al., 2014). Subsequently, research has demonstrated the benefits, participant retention rate, and cost-effectiveness of a choir programme of high-intensity singing, vocal exercises, and daily home practice for people with Parkinson's (Matthews, 2018). An Australian study ("ParkinSong") also found significant improvements in some voice measures (vocal intensity and maximum expiratory pressure; Tamplin et al., 2019). An international study of the Sing To Beat Parkinson's programme found psychosocial benefits and improved social support for people living with Parkinson's but did not include voice measures (Irons et al., 2020). Each study protocol varies in detail, but all focus on regular (usually weekly) sessions incorporating a welcome, warm-ups and breathing exercises, a sustained period of song-singing, and usually a social time with refreshments and conversation. Participation may be maximised through physical, respiration and voice exercises, thoughtful selection of songs, and attention to musical elements, such as regular metres, rhythmic regularity, predominantly stepwise melodic contour, and contrasting tempi and dynamics (Buetow et al., 2013; Matthews et al., 2019).

Dementia

> I may not remember everything, everyone,
> Everywhere I've been,
> I may not remember everything,
> But I'm still me.
>
> *(Talmage, 2020e)*

Dementia is a family of neurological conditions in which changes in the brain cause a gradual loss of functioning in the acts of daily living. The international prevalence of dementia, around 50 million, is expected to rise to 152 million by 2050 (Alzheimer's Disease International, 2019). People with late-stage Parkinson's may also experience dementia, and some forms of dementia (such as primary progressive aphasia) initially affect language and communication. Dementia gradually but severely limits communication, daily activities, and the quality of relationships. Musical responsiveness is more robust, with the ability to enjoy listening to music and singing often surviving when other skills are lost – as in my case study of Florence (Talmage, 2018a).

Researchers have studied singing groups for people living with dementia, led by trained facilitators (Osman et al., 2016) or by music therapists (Clark et al., 2018). The findings of both studies emphasised themes of inclusion, support, friendship, personal relationships, and a sense of well-being. The proportion of CeleBRation Choir participants living with dementia has increased in recent years, due to peer recommendations in dementia support groups. Two members are instrumentalists, sustaining their musical skills by playing in the choir's band – another future research topic.

Choir programme

> Our study showed people will take part,
> And test their voices at the start,
> In the middle of term and before they depart,
> Oh, we all love the CeleBRation Choir!
> *(Talmage et al., 2013, p. 47)*

The success of New Zealand's neurological choirs demonstrates a demand for this approach. Successful participant recruitment in several research studies illustrates members' eagerness to contribute to knowledge creation, best practice, and equity.

Our repertoire is selected in collaboration with the members. Favourite songs include popular music from past decades, cultural songs, show tunes, and a few classical and jazz numbers. In a large group of people with an age range of 40 to 90 years, we foster tolerance of others' preferences and a 'give it a go' attitude. Humour and positive lyrics keep spirits up, but tender emotions and sad memories are not avoided. Given participant demographics, bereavements are not uncommon and are always acknowledged through singing and shared stories. Familiar songs often elicit reminiscence, and by singing them together and for others, the choir is also creating new memories.

Mumbled complaints about vocal exercise have prompted me to transform exercises into songs! Melody, rhythm, lyrics, and song structure may achieve greater engagement and enjoyment than repetitive drills. For example, "We Just Wanna Sing!" (Figure 8.2) includes sustained phonation (bar 1), rhythmic speech patterns, vocables that emphasise articulation, and a reduced cognitive load of word production.

Physical warm-ups and posture are also addressed through song. "Get Ready to Sing!" (Figure 8.3) is a call-and-copy action song that draws attention from feet to head, one verse at a time.

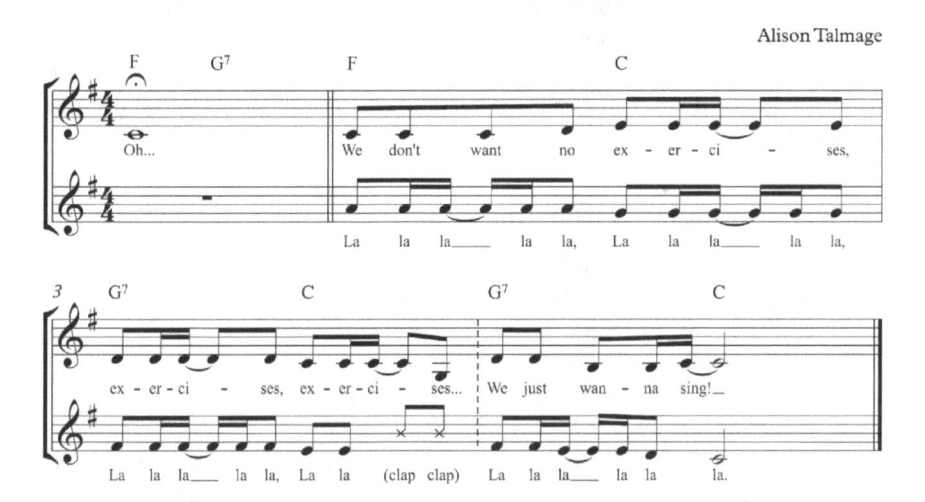

Figure 8.2 "We Just Wanna Sing!" (extract; Talmage, 2018b)

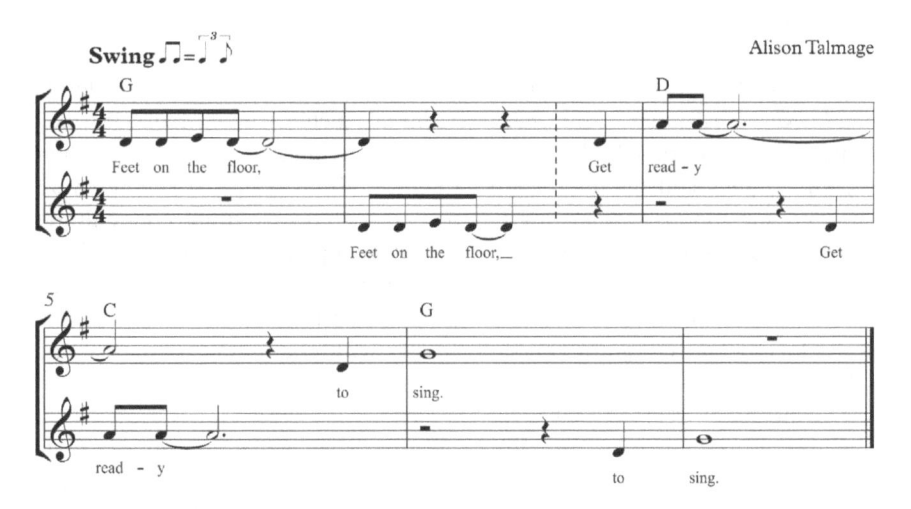

Figure 8.3 "Get Ready to Sing!" Warm-up song composed for the choir (extract; Talmage, 2020a)

Our song-leading style differs from regular community choirs. Simplified gestures are more helpful than formal conducting skills. Leading by singing is more common than in formal choirs, and much is conveyed through general body language, facial expressions, and varied proximity to the singers. I usually accompany the choir on the guitar, which allows me to move around, and suits much of the popular music repertoire. Sometimes I play the piano, violin, or drum along with our ad hoc band of volunteers and two members living with dementia. Many choirs separate the conductor and accompanist roles, but playing enables more direct control of tempo, style, rubato, and spontaneous playfulness rather than singing on automatic pilot. I relish those magic moments when the music flows, and I can step back from my facilitator role and become just another participant.

Enablers and barriers to participation

> Songs from your culture help you sing along,
> Though travelling far makes it harder for some,
> If you have a carer who is ready to come,
> Oh, you will love the CeleBRation Choir!
> *(Talmage et al., 2013, p. 48)*

In an ideal world, all communities would offer accessible community choirs and rehabilitation services. For people living with a neurological condition, mobility and transport issues often prevent independent participation. However, the choir is also enriched by the participation of companions who often provide transport.

Cultural factors may play a significant part in whether people may choose to join the choir. Past and present CeleBRation Choir members are predominantly New Zealanders of European descent but include some Māori, Pasifika, Indian, and Asian people. We listen to what individuals need, welcome their support people, and discuss their song choices. Individually and collectively, choir participation is enriched by singing alongside people from other cultures and working collaboratively to share (without appropriating) their music. However, mainstream popular music, a significant part of our repertoire, may be less familiar to older people whose first language is not English. Future approaches could include collaboration and skill-sharing with community musicians and other professionals.

During New Zealand's COVID-19 lockdowns, the CeleBRation Choir met online, with a focus on singing, songwriting, and peer support (Talmage, 2020c; Talmage et al., 2020). Although technology and the online environment were not accessible to all members, feedback from attendees was very positive. The challenge of physical distancing and coping strategies were expressed through song selection, such as this adaptation of a traditional round, "Hey Ho!" (Figure 8.4), which led to collaborative songwriting projects. Contact with those unable to participate online was sustained through phone calls, email, and offering audio and video resources for use at home.

The common thread is community: the choir as a community within a wider community and the wider community support needed for sustainable practice.

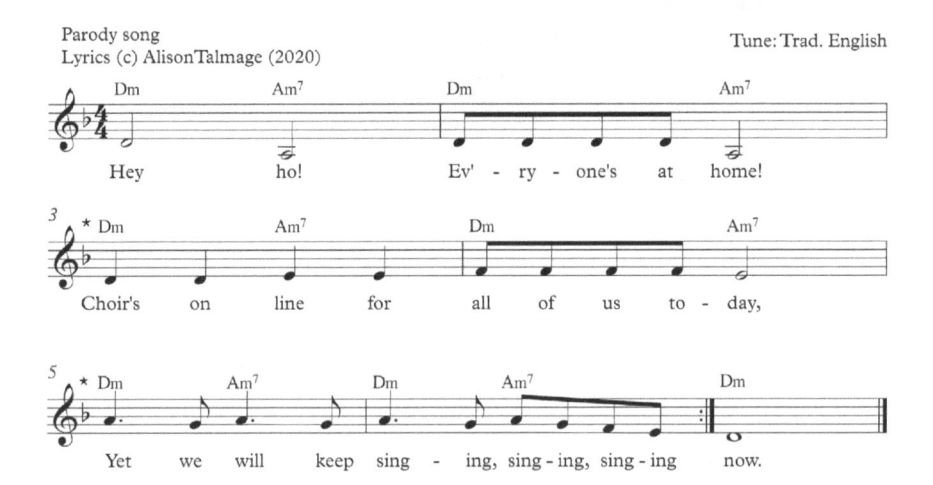

Figure 8.4 "Hey Ho!" (parody song; Talmage, 2020b)

Coda: a neurological choir manifesto

Our choir members recognise one another's struggles with communication and sense of loss. A sense of belonging is perhaps the choir's greatest drawcard. Together, participants are empowered to vocalise and sing; request, create, or refuse songs; and advocate for others facing similar challenges. Both peer support and the allyship of non-disabled supporters are needed.

Singing – as an opportunity for self-expression – is a human right. The Universal Declaration of Human Rights includes, in Article 27, "the right freely to participate in the cultural life of the community, to enjoy the arts and to share in scientific advancement and its benefits" and, in Article 19, "the right to freedom of opinion and expression" (United Nations, 1948). As a music therapist, I have an ethical obligation to advocate for service provision that empowers people to lead fulfilling lives in their families and communities.

Researchers have called for more robust study designs, enabling meta-analysis of programmes and outcomes (Dingle et al., 2019). However, within music therapy a tension exists between ecological, exploratory, collaborative approaches (Denora & Ansdell, 2017) and calls for strict protocol fidelity in randomised controlled trials (Baker et al., 2019). In my current doctoral study, I am approaching practice improvement through action research – developing guidelines that foreground the voices, experiences, and aspirations of people living with disability and honour the CBR's aim of working together to improve lives.

Acknowledgements

I would like to thank past and present members of the CeleBRation Choir; my doctoral supervisors at the University of Auckland, Professor Suzanne Purdy and Dr Te Oti Rakena; and at Te Herenga Waka – Victoria University of Wellington, Associate Professor Daphne Rickson. I would also like to thank the Centre for Brain Research, particularly Distinguished Professor Sir Richard Faull; University of Auckland advisers, Dr Clare McCann and Dr Anna Miles; and past and present clinical supervisors, Claire Molyneux and Liz Wallace.

References

Alzheimer's Disease International. (2019). *World Alzheimer's report 2019: Attitudes to dementia.* www.alz.co.uk/research/world-report-2019

Baker, F. A., Tamplin, J., Clark, I. N., Lee, Y.-E. C., Geretsegger, M., & Gold, C. (2019). Treatment fidelity in a music therapy multi-site cluster randomised controlled trial for people living with dementia: The MIDDEL project intervention fidelity protocol. *Journal of Music Therapy, 56*(2), 125–148. https://doi.org/10.1093/jmt/thy023

Brady, M. C., Kelly, H., Godwin, J., Enderby, P., & Campbell, P. (2016). Speech and language therapy for aphasia following stroke. *Cochrane Database of Systematic Reviews 2016, 6,* Article CD000425. https://doi.org/10.1002/14651858.CD000425.pub4

Buetow, S., Talmage, A., McCann, C., Fogg, L., & Purdy, S. (2013). Conceptualising how group singing may enhance quality of life with Parkinson's disease. *Disability & Rehabilitation, 36*(5), 430–433. doi:10.3109/09638288.2013.793749

CeleBRation Choir. (2020). *In our own words – Why we all love the CeleBRation Choir* [Video file]. University of Auckland. www.facebook.com/CeleBRationChoirNZ/videos/1737677036401922/

Chadha, S. (Director). (2019). *Sing, they all said, just sing. YouTube* [Film]. www.youtube.com/watch?v=kqn9yup4A_g&feature=youtu.be

Christian, D. (2016, December 10). Singing the praises of choirs. *New Zealand Herald.* www.nzherald.co.nz/dionne-christian/news/article.cfm?a_id=1048&objectid=11764026

Clark, I. N., Tamplin, J. D., & Baker, F. A. (2018). Community-dwelling people living with dementia and their family caregivers experience enhanced relationships and feelings of well-being following therapeutic group singing: A qualitative thematic analysis. *Frontiers in Psychology, 9.* https://doi.org/10.3389/fpsyg.2018.01332

Dashtipour, K., Tafreshi, A., Lee, J., & Crawley, B. (2018). Speech disorders in Parkinson's disease: Pathophysiology, medical management and surgical approaches. *Neurodegenerative Disease Management, 8*(5), 337–348. https://doi.org/10.2217/nmt-2018-0021

Daveson, B. (2008). A description of a music therapy meta-model in neuro-disability and neuro-rehabilitation for use with children, adolescents and adults. *Australian Journal of Music Therapy, 19.* www.austmta.org.au/journal/search?issue=833&query=

Denora, T., & Ansdell, G. (2017). Music in action: Tinkering, testing and tracing over time. *Qualitative Research, 17*(2), 231–245. https://doi.org/10.1177/1468794116682824

Di Benedetto, P., Cavazzon, M., Mondolo, F., Rugiu, G., Peratoner, A., & Biasutti, E. (2009a). Voice and choral singing treatment: A new approach for speech and voice disorders in Parkinson's disease. *European Journal of Physical and Rehabilitation Medicine, 45*(1), 13–19.

Dingle, G. A., Clift, S., Finn, S., Gilbert, R., Groarke, J. M., Irons, J. Y., Bartoli, A. J., Lamont, A., Launay, J., Martin, E. S., Talbot, S., Tarrant, M., Tip, L., & Williams, E. J. (2019). An agenda for best practice research on group singing, health, and well-being. *Music & Science, 2*, 1–15. https://doi.org/10.1177/2059204319861719

Durie, M. H. (1985). A Maori perspective of health. *Social Science & Medicine, 20*, 483–486. https://doi.org/10.1016/0277-9536(85)90363-6

Fogg-Rogers, L., Buetow, S., Talmage, A., McCann, C. M., Leão, S. H. S., Tippett, L., Leung, J., McPherson, K. M., & Purdy, S. C. (2016). Choral singing therapy following stroke or Parkinson's disease: An exploration of participants' experiences. *Disability and Rehabilitation, 38*(10), 952–962. https://doi.org/10.3109/09638288.2015.1068875

GBD 2019 Diseases and Injuries Collaborators. (2020). Stroke – Level 3 cause. In global burden of 369 diseases and injuries in 204 countries and territories, 1990–2019: A systematic analysis for the global burden of disease study 2019. *The Lancet, 396*, https://doi.org/10.1016/S0140-6736(20)30925-9

Hatala, A. R. (2013). Towards a biopsychosocial – spiritual approach in health psychology: Exploring theoretical orientations and future directions. *Journal of Spirituality in Mental Health, 15*(4), 256–276.

Hicks, R. (2018). Just sing! In C. Molyneux (Ed.), *Tales from the music therapy room: Creative connections* (pp. 124–125). Jessica Kingsley.

Irons, J. Y., Hancox, G., Vella-Burrows, T., Han, E.-Y., Chong, H. J., Sheffield, D., & Stewart, D. E. (2020). Group singing improves quality of life for people with Parkinson's: An international study. *Aging & Mental Health*. https://doi.org/10.1080/13607863.2020.1720599

Jenkins, B., Storie, S., & Purdy, S. C. (2017). Quality of life for individuals with a neurological condition who participate in social/therapeutic choirs. *New Zealand Journal of Music Therapy, 15*, 59–94.

Johnston, R. (2019, May 24). Joys of choir singing change Aucklander's life for the better after major stroke at age 32. *New Zealand Herald*. www.nzherald.co.nz/lifestyle/news/article.cfm?c_id=6&objectid=12215005

Koelsch, S. (2012). Toward a neural basis of music perception – A review and updated model. *Frontiers in Psychology, 2*, 110. https://doi.org/10.3389/fpsyg.2011.00110

Martinez-Martin, P., Chaudhuri, K. R., Rojo-Abuin, J. M., Rodriguez-Blazquez, C., Alvarez-Sanchez, M., Arakaki, T., Bergareche-Yarza, A., Chade, A., Garretto, N., Gershanik, O., Kurtis, M. M., Mendoza-Rodriguez, A., Moore, H. P., Rodriguez-Violante, M., Singer, C., Tilley, B. C., Huang, J., Stebbins, G. T., & Goetz, C. G. (2015). Assessing the non-motor symptoms of Parkinson's disease: MDS - UPDRS and NMS scale. *European Journal of Neurology, 22*(1), 37–43. https://doi:10.1111/ene.12165

Matthews, R. M. (2018). *Acoustic, respiratory, cognitive and wellbeing comparisons of two groups of people with Parkinson's disease participating in voice and choral singing group therapy (VCST) versus a music appreciation activity* (Unpublished doctoral thesis). University of Auckland. https://researchspace.auckland.ac.nz/handle/2292/37599

Matthews, R. M., Purdy, S. C., & Tippett, L. J. (2019). Song choice and vocal exercises in group singing for people with Parkinson's disease: The perspective of a speech- language therapist/musician. *New Zealand Journal of Music Therapy, 17*, 25–40. www.musictherapy.org.nz/journal/2019-2

Music Therapy New Zealand. (2019). *Music therapy: Connecting communities* [Video file]. www.facebook.com/1025218250854404/videos/241236146763621

Osman, S. E., Tischler, V., & Schneider, J. (2016). "Singing for the brain": A qualitative study exploring the health and well-being benefits of singing for people with dementia and their carers. *Dementia, 15*(6), 1326–1339. https://doi.org/10.1177/1471301214556291

Purdy, S. C. (2020). Communication research in the context of *te whare tapa whā* model of health. *International Journal of Speech-Language Pathology, 22*(3), 281–289. https://doi.org/10.1080/17549507.2020.1768288

Radio New Zealand. (2013). *2013: A medley of songs by the CeleBRation choir* [Audio file]. www.rnz.co.nz/national/programmes/nat-music/audio/2573528/2013-a-medley-of-songs-by-the-celebration-choir

Rickson, D. (2012, November). Music therapy New Zealand conference 2012 – "Music and the brain: Developing pathways". *MusT: A Newsletter from Music Therapy New Zealand, 406.* www.musictherapy.org.nz/wp-content/uploads/2018/10/MusT-November-2012.pdf

Sapir, S. (2014). Multiple factors are involved in the dysarthria associated with Parkinson's disease: A review with implications for clinical practice and research (report). *Journal of Speech, Language, and Hearing Research, 57*(4), 1330. https://doi.org/10.1044/2014_JSLHR-S-13-0039

Särkämö, T., & Sihvonen, A. J. (2018). Golden oldies and silver brains: Deficits, preservation, learning, and rehabilitation effects of music in ageing-related neurological disorders. *Cortex, 109,* 104–123. https://doi.org/10.1016/j.cortex.2018.08.034

Stahl, B., Kotz, S. A., Helseler, I., Turner, R., & Geyer, S. (2011). Rhythm in disguise: Why singing may not hold the key to recovery from aphasia. *Brain, 134*(10), 3083–3093. https://doi.org/10.1093/brain/awr240

Talmage, A. (2018a). Florence. In C. Molyneux (Ed.), *Tales from the music therapy room: Creative connections* (pp. 118–122). Jessica Kingsley. (Original work published 2017).

Talmage, A. (2018b). *We just Wanna sing.* [Musical score]. CeleBRation Choir. https://celebrationchoirnews.wordpress.com/songs

Talmage, A. (2020a). *Get ready to sing.* [Musical score]. CeleBRation Choir. https://celebrationchoirnews.wordpress.com/songs

Talmage, A. (2020b). *Hey Ho!* [Musical score]. CeleBRation Choir. https://celebrationchoirnews.wordpress.com/songs

Talmage, A. (2020c). Log on and sing: Songwriting with the CeleBRation Choir. In A. Talmage, M. B. C. Clulee, H. Cho, M. Glass, J. Gordon, S. Hoskyns, B. J. Hunt, A. A. H. Jeong, L. Johns, J. C. Kong, E. Langlois Hunt, E. Matthews, D. Rickson, C. Riegelhaupt Landreani, S. Sabri, & R. Solly (Eds.), *Music therapy in a time of pandemic: Experiences of musicking, telehealth, and resource-oriented practice during COVID-19 in Aotearoa New Zealand* (pp. 50–54). *New Zealand Journal of Music Therapy, 18,* 7–66. www.musictherapy.org.nz/journal/2020-2

Talmage, A. (2020d). *Singing all together.* [Musical score]. CeleBRation Choir. https://celebrationchoirnews.wordpress.com/songs

Talmage, A. (2020e). *Still me.* [Musical score]. CeleBRation Choir. https://celebrationchoirnews.wordpress.com/songs

Talmage, A., Fogg-Rogers, L., Leão, S. H. S., & Purdy, S. C. (2014). Choral singing therapy for a client with Parkinson's disease. In C. Miller (Ed.), *Assessment and outcomes in the arts therapies: A person-centred approach* (pp. 54–66). Jessica Kingsley.

Talmage, A., Ludlam, S., Leão, S., Fogg-Rogers, L., & Purdy, S. (2013). Leading the CeleBRation Choir: The choral singing therapy protocol and the role of the music therapist in a social singing group for adults with neurological conditions. *New Zealand Journal of Music Therapy, 11,* 7–50.

Talmage, A., Purdy, S., Rakena, T., & Rickson, D. (2020, May*). "Choir online is better than no choir at all!" Responses of adults with neurological conditions to an e-choir initiative during Covid-19 lockdown in New Zealand.* Poster presentation for the Brain. Cognition. Emotion. Music. Conference (BCEM), University of Kent, UK. https://osf.io/yctj7

Tamplin, J., Baker, F. A., Jones, B., Way, A., & Stuart, L. (2013). "Stroke a chord": The effect of singing in a community choir on mood and social engagement for people living with aphasia following a stroke. *Neurorehabilitation, 32*(4), 929–941.

Tamplin, J., Morris, M. E., Marigliani, C., Baker, F. A., & Vogel, A. P. (2019). ParkinSong: A controlled trial of singing-based therapy for Parkinson's disease. *Neurorehabilitation and Neural Repair, 33*(6), 453–463. https://doi.org/10.1177/1545968319847948

Thompson, N., Storie, S., & Purdy, S. (2017). "Catching the tune or channelling the beat": A pilot study investigating the role of rhythm in therapeutic singing for aphasia. *New Zealand Journal of Music Therapy, 15*, 122–161.

TVNZ. (2016, May 22). Singing the remedy of choice for choir members with neurological conditions. *One News.* www.tvnz.co.nz/one-news/new-zealand/singing-remedy-choice-choir-members-neurological-conditions

United Nations. (1948). *Universal declaration of human rights.* www.un.org/en/about-us/universal-declaration-of-human-rights

Ward, L., & Cannon, M. (2018). A patient-centred approach to stroke prevention. *Practice Nursing, 29*(7). https://doi-org.ezproxy.auckland.ac.nz/10.12968/pnur.2018.29.7.316

West, S. (2009). Selective Mutism for Singing (SMS) and its treatment: Conceptualising musical disengagement as mass social dysfunction. In W. Baker (Ed.), *Proceedings of the Australian society for music education XVII conference* (pp. 212–220). University of Tasmania.

White, M. (2018, Spring). The power of voice. *Ingenico: The University of Auckland Alumni Magazine,* 28–29. www.auckland.ac.nz/content/dam/uoa/alumni/publications/ingenio/Ingenio-Spring-2018.pdf

Worrall, L. E., Hudson, K., Khan, A., Brooke, R., & Simmons-Mackie, N. (2017). Determinants of living well with aphasia in the first year poststroke: A prospective cohort study. *Archives of Physical Medicine and Rehabilitation, 98*(2), 235–240. https://doi.org/10.1016/j.apmr.2016.06.020

Zumbansen, A., Peretz, I., & Hébert, S. (2014). The combination of rhythm and pitch can account for the beneficial effect of melodic intonation therapy on connected speech improvements in Broca's aphasia. *Frontiers in Human Neuroscience, 8*, 592. https://doi.org/10.3389/fnhum.2014.00592

9 Music therapy for autistic children – responding to contemporary understandings with new research approaches

Daphne Rickson

Introduction

Autism spectrum disorder

Autism spectrum disorder (ASD) is an umbrella medical term used to describe a diverse group of developmental conditions that affect people's ability to relate to and communicate with neurotypical people. It is characterised by core features including difficulties with social communication and interaction and restricted interests and/or repetitive behaviours (American Psychiatric Association, 2013). Estimates suggest one in 160 children worldwide (World Health Organisation, 2019) is diagnosed with the condition, highlighting the need for research that supports management and/or promotes understanding.

There is already a significant body of medical research which aims to highlight neurological causality for the symptoms associated with ASD. However, studies have provided inconsistent evidence, due to small sample sizes, differences in participant characteristics such as age, and the heterogeneity of ASD (Khundrakpam et al., 2017; Waterhouse et al., 2016). Waterhouse et al. (2016) argue that "no unitary brain impairment theory to date has been replicated to become a standard explanation of ASD brain disruption" (p. 303). They further suggest that while the diagnosis is important for explaining a child's way of being and introducing them to an early behavioural intervention, research has not yet uncovered diagnosis-specific medical treatment, a consistent early predictor, or a unified life course.

Medicine has highlighted a myriad of 'deficiencies' or 'abnormalities' associated with ASD that are presumed to prevent people who have this 'disorder' from participating fully and meaningfully within their communities. Through this 'medical model of disability' lens, it is assumed that people with ASD want to be different, to be other than as they are, to be cured (Swain & French, 2000). However, disability is now seen as the result of complex interactions among biological, psychological, cultural, and socio-political factors (Anastasiou & Kauffman, 2012). Advocates of the 'biopsychosocial model of disability' recognise that autism is underpinned by biological differences but also see it

DOI: 10.4324/9781003082897-13

as an important and natural human variation (Baker, 2010; Kapp et al., 2013; Ne'eman, 2010).

Baron-Cohen (2017) argues genetic, neural, behavioural, and cognitive evidence suggests that autistic people are different, and may live with a disability but not a disorder. He suggests that "disability requires societal support, acceptance of difference and diversity, and societal 'reasonable adjustment', whilst disorder is usually taken to require cure or treatment" (p. 745). The 'affirmative model of disability' takes this further, offering a non-tragic view of disability and impairment which encompasses positive individual and collective social identities for disabled people (Swain & French, 2000) and recognises that disability can be valuable, exciting, and intrinsically satisfying (Campbell, 2008). In this chapter, the term *autistic children* is used as a positive identity marker (Evans, 2018).

The heterogeneity of autism provides legitimacy for multiple agendas. Importantly, neurodiversity and disability rights advocates have expressed acceptance of informed choice regarding identity, prevention, and cure (Kapp et al., 2013). Empathic collaboration between researchers and communities can help people to make informed choices that attend to the rights, responsibilities, and social and political needs of all parties (Baker, 2010).

Music therapy practice

Music has been used to support the well-being of autistic people for a very long time (Reschke-Hernandez, 2011). Music therapists have used a range of developmental, relational, interactive, music, psychoanalytic, and neurologically based approaches to address a variety of non-musical or music-centred goals (Bergmann, 2016). Their methods include improvisation, receptive methods, the use of pre-composed music, and/or song writing. Despite this diversity, music therapy programmes with autistic children typically focus on developing communication, social interaction, and emotional expression, and improvisation is the main method used (Bergmann, 2016; Geretsegger et al., 2015; Wigram & Gold, 2006).

The improvisational approach is relationship-based, grounded in the child's ability to attend, adapt, and engage with their own and others' musical play (Carpente & LaGasse, 2014; Geretsegger et al., 2015; Slootsky & Gold, 2016). It provides children with a means to express, communicate, and interact, and to develop socioemotional functioning. That is, the core features of ASD, relating and communicating, are addressed through a process involving the music therapist and child engaging in collaborative music-making and managing the roles, relationships, and dynamics that emerge (Bergmann, 2016; Carpente & LaGasse, 2014; Geretsegger et al., 2015; Slootsky & Gold, 2016; Wimpory & Gwilym, 2019).

Autistic people can have significant cognitive strengths, particularly attention and memory for detail and a strong drive to detect patterns or 'systemising' (Baron-Cohen, 2017). They often have an affinity for music and may exhibit special musical abilities (Heaton, 2004; Janzen & Thaut, 2018), including intact or superior music processing abilities in the areas of pitch, timbre, melodic memory, the rules of Western musical harmony, and rhythm synchronisation (Janzen & Thaut, 2018). Many have exceptionally good pitch information processing skills including the rare ability to identify or produce the pitch of a tone without external reference (Janzen & Thaut, 2018). Music is therefore engaging and motivating for many and has high potential as a therapeutic medium. Bakan (2018) writes of 'Donald', for example, who found music to be "a welcome refuge from the interpersonal engagements of the outside world" and of 'Graeme' who used it as an essential bridge to social relationships "linking him deeply to people [in the music world] he might otherwise have never gotten to know".

Improvisational music therapy research

Research investigating improvisational music therapy to improve social communication skills, self-awareness, and emotional expression and understanding of autistic children has produced promising results (Geretsegger et al., 2014; James et al., 2015; Janzen & Thaut, 2018). A systematic review of 10 clinical trials found moderate to large effects of music therapy on social interaction, non-verbal communication, social-emotional reciprocity, and parent–child relationship, suggesting music therapy may address the core of the ASD condition (Geretsegger et al., 2014). However, a more recent large-scale multi-centre randomised clinical trial (RCT), involving 364 children aged between 4 and 7 years, did not support these results (Bieleninik et al., 2017). Bieleninik et al. (2017) compared improvisational music therapy with enhanced standard care over a period of five months and found no significant difference in symptom severity based on the Autism Diagnostic Observation Schedule (ADOS) social affect domain.

Examining the potential reasons behind contradictory results is particularly important because RCTs and meta-analyses are considered the most rigorous forms of positivist research (Broder-Fingert et al., 2017). The inconsistent findings may be explained by variations in local contexts, the numbers of therapists involved in the studies, variations in implementation of improvisational interventions, inconsistent attendance of participants, the choice of proximal versus a distal outcome, and the ADOS as a measurement tool (Bieleninik et al., 2017). The age range of the children was narrow (4–7 years), but they hailed from nine different countries; had experienced various linguistic, musical, and other cultural backgrounds; and had various levels of intellectual ability. When results are averaged across such a heterogeneous population the potential to demonstrate differences is reduced. Studies included in Geretsegger et al. (2014) meta-analysis were also considered to be heterogeneous and overall, of moderate to low quality.

Rationale for new forms of research

Music therapy is a small field capable of meeting a comprehensive range of objectives for an extremely wide range of services users (McFerran & Silverman, 2018). Research is crucial to enable the delivery of safe and positive outcomes and thus to the success of the profession. However, complex political and organisational contexts influence the type of research that is conducted and/ or drawn on in any situation (McFerran & Silverman, 2018). For example, in many contemporary music therapy contexts in which health and well-being are recognised as sociocultural processes the positivist bias and hierarchical nature of 'levels of evidence' within evidence-based practice (EBP) make it extremely problematic (Aigen, 2015; Borgnakke, 2017; Edwards, 2005; Else & Wheeler, 2010; Otera, 2013; Rickson et al., 2016; Silverman, 2010; Wheeler & Bruscia, 2016). Policymakers and practitioners are increasingly aware of the limitations of RCTs and the value of interpretivist evidence for informing and judging the quality of EBP (Aigen, 2015; Kinn et al., 2013; Rickson et al., 2016).

Music therapists accept the need to engage with EBP in order to make appropriate decisions within their music therapy practices. However, the reduction of complexity, which is fundamental to RCTs and other positivist designs, can result in profound loss of meaning and relevance in real-world contexts (Edwards, 2002, 2005). Instead, we need to stay close to our experiences, remain pragmatic, and "reject rigid, abstract rules of what constitutes knowledge" (Aigen, 2015, p. 33). Aigen (2015) notes the things that matter most to music therapists are that participants, family members, and other professionals are satisfied with music therapy; that it has benefits for participants that can also be seen by institutions, agencies, and communities where it is offered; and, finally, whether it works as a treatment modality (Aigen, 2015, p. 15). The involvement of end users in the research process is therefore becoming increasingly important (Geretsegger, 2019).

Participants in exploratory research examining music therapy with children who have ASD in New Zealand (Rickson et al., 2016) expressed strong interest in research focusing on the ways parents, teachers, other professionals, as well as people with ASD, perceive the music therapy process, and stressed that their voices should be included where possible. This prompted the project described below, which focuses on the way teams of 'evaluators' perceived autistic children's involvement in music therapy.

The perceived value of music therapy for autistic children

The research involved a multiple case study design to investigate the perceived impact of music therapy in supporting the interpersonal communication of autistic children (Rickson, 2021). Ten registered music therapists each delivered individual music therapy sessions to an autistic child who had not experienced music therapy before, mostly weekly, for up to one year. Practice evidence was captured via video, descriptions of music therapy interactions, feedback from parents and other professionals, and/or from other clinical tools that music therapists might choose to use. They used this material to develop a case report of their work, which they submitted to the researcher in the form of "narrative assessment" (Carr, 2001).

The case reports, or narrative assessments, contained at least three "learning stories" (Carr, 2001). Learning stories are short accounts of participant learning presented in a consistent form. They include descriptions of the participant's character, an introduction to the setting in which the learning took place, detailed accounts of key interactions to give a rich context to the progress being described, and a summary and reflection on what the story or stories demonstrated. In the study described here, the music therapists' summaries and reflections were produced on separate documents and withheld from evaluators. Photographs and video were used to complement and clarify the story.

Data gathering and analysis

The music therapists' rich interpretivist case reports were not treated as data, but artefacts to be examined, with informed consent from all parties, by teams of evaluators (made up of several people who knew the child and six independent autism experts who did not). The six independent experts, who had multiple expertise as parents, teachers of typical and diverse populations, a member of an ASD disability action group, an education lecturer, a psychologist, an autism advisor, a policy analyst, and an autistic adult, evaluated all 10 cases. The evaluators provided 85 descriptive evaluations and completed 86 Likert questionnaires to communicate their understanding of whether, how, and why music therapy might have a positive or negative effect on the child.

The researcher (author) developed a thematic analysis of each case and drew descriptive statistics from the positivist findings, to determine how the music therapy processes were understood and valued by people who knew one of the children, and by independent experts who did not know the children. Further analysis enabled themes from all 10 cases to be compared to determine the ways music therapy was perceived overall and to discover whether, and in what ways, music therapy was perceived similarly or differently according to the position/lens of the observer.

In the following vignette describing evaluators' perceptions of 'Liam's' case and the brief overview of the wider findings, people who knew the child are identified by their relationship to Liam, while independent autism experts have been given nom de plumes.

Case vignette

Background

Liam was 8 years old and a bright, talkative child. However, he had difficulty listening and concentrating and was often described as being 'in his own world'. He loved to sing but not in front of other people. His challenges with interpersonal communication meant that it was hard for him to make friends. Jodie, his music therapist, employed a child-centred approach, following Liam's lead when planning and facilitating the sessions. Their work together spanned 14 sessions over a five-month period.

The learning stories described three contrasting activities. In the first, the pair were engaged in a playful sleep/wake game with Jodie pretending to sleep and Liam waking her up with a 'boo'! When Jodie improvised a song about the activity, Liam, who had been upset on arrival, danced joyfully around the room requesting more. In the second example, Liam was sharing his session with his cousin and making a CD of his singing to share with others. He was communicating his choice of musical materials, as well as ideas for the cover of his CD. In the final example, Liam was improvising at the keyboard with Jodie. Prior to this session, while he enjoyed playing, he had preferred to play on his own. In this session, he was able to engage in several exchanges of musical turn taking.

Evaluators' observations of Liam at music therapy

> *Liam is twirling in space (a favourite of autistic kids as it can be soothing) but when the music stops; he joins in the game of waking up the therapist (by saying 'boo'!). Playing such an interactive game requires imagination, and suggests to me that Liam is enjoying the learning that is taking place.*
>
> *(Hilda)*

The evaluators noticed how much Liam enjoyed the sessions, and how they opened opportunities for him to learn and develop. Family members shared that Liam played the 'boo' game at home and believed that he introduced it to music therapy as a strategy to help him overcome his anxiety. His use of humour helped him regulate his emotions.

Evaluators were particularly impressed with Liam's spontaneous participation at the keyboard. They saw his confidence clearly developing over time; especially in terms of allowing himself to be heard (he was eventually able to sing in front of others). His improvisations became increasingly dynamic and creative. He began to 'experiment' with sounds, to purposefully seek out notes.

> *Although at the start Liam played some quite basic notes (on the piano), as he progressed and gained more confidence it sounded more tuneful and expressive. I thought it interesting that he tried to play a melody rather than crashing on the keyboard. I loved the very confident improvised scale at the end.*
>
> *(Grandmother)*

However, evaluators also noticed that while Liam was enthusiastic and eager to play, he was also able to keep time and to wait his turn. They could see that he was aware that he needed to consider Jodie's needs and feelings and was exercising patience. He was acutely attentive, concentrating on and planning what he would play in response to her music.

> *Children with ASD often have difficulty waiting their turn and while they can be rule driven, it is not unusual for them to become frustrated. It was good to see that the turns were of different durations and in some instances Liam clearly thought it was his turn and was about to jump in and then held himself back. He had great concentration and it was a pleasure to be able to see the connection between him and his therapist.*
>
> *(Freya)*

Evaluators noted how Jodie was able to develop a repertoire of opportunities which appealed to Liam and kept him engaged. He was 'at ease with her' and his genuine engagement, and increasing collaboration, demonstrated that he trusted her. He was observed to develop a strong connection with her over the course of the therapy.

Family members reported that in his early years, Liam had been distressed by loud noises. His aunt and grandmother were therefore impressed with how 'conditioned' to noise he seemed at music therapy and his enjoyment of playing the cymbal. His passion and appreciation for music, his 'natural musicality', and his musical abilities were mentioned frequently by evaluators; and music was said to be a very appropriate therapeutic medium for him.

> *This case demonstrates that for those children with autism who have a natural flair for music in combination with an intuitive therapist, can be a win–win combination for increasing specific competencies that can be generalised by students to their learn- ing and social settings*
>
> *(Vivian)*

Liam was also observed to be using reasoning and judgement when working on his recording project, watching and learning from his cousin. It was evident that even during this one session, his ability to make choices improved. Evalua- tors could therefore see opportunities not only for developing Liam's interest in music further but also for developing relationships with others who share this interest. Mike, who has lived experience of autism, argued that Liam's social skills developed 'as much as could reasonably be expected for an 8-year-old in this short but sustained period'. Hilda and Ruella suggested that while it was a good idea to have individual sessions initially, more might have been achieved if peers were involved in an ongoing way.

Brief overview of wider findings

The findings from Liam's case resonate with those from the wider study. Eval- uators strongly believed that music therapy was important for nine of the 10 children involved, while in the outlying case the introduction of medication led to disagreement regarding the cause of the positive change (Rickson, 2021). They observed that in music therapy, children were able to express themselves musically, verbally, and/or physically and were engaged in meaningful interaction. Music and dance offered an important alternative means of communication for them. The rhythms and patterns of music seemed to help them to feel safe, and the 'attunement' and 'synchronisation' that occurred as part of the musical relationship contributed significantly to the establishment of rapport.

The music therapists employed child-centred and/or music-centred approaches, which enabled learning and development to happen in natural ways. The evaluators observed that they were intuitive, ingenious, creative, and patient therapists and musicians who readily developed secure therapeutic relationships with the children. An important aspect of the work was the music therapists' abilities to balance flexibility and spontaneity with predictability and familiarity, as needed. Sensory input was incorporated into the sessions according to the children's needs.

The children were readily engaged and increasingly able to focus. Individuals variously began to look for communicative cues from others, and to move from fleeting moments of connection to sustained periods of playful interaction. Each of the children demonstrated increases in their cognitive skills, either beginning or increasing their abilities to attend, listen, concentrate, wait, turn take, share, express preferences and make choices, take initiatives, negotiate, and/or follow instructions. Some were able to engage in problem-solving and other related cognitive tasks and to demonstrate increases in expressive language, including speech. Music therapy was seen to lessen children's stress, anxiety, frustration, and need to maintain control, enabling them to share a range of emotions in safe and acceptable ways. Some began to tolerate imperfection, take risks and try new things, learn to consider the perspectives of others, compromise, and negotiate.

Their critical analysis of the case studies enabled families and others who knew the children to see them interacting in unexpected ways. And, despite acknowledging the music therapists' considerable expertise, evaluators also recognised strategies that could be used at home, and in schools to help facilitate individual education plans. Nevertheless, for some children, the importance of individual support was emphasised with the therapeutic space being described as "a little oasis of positive one-on-one therapy that is enjoyable and sensory in a positive way without any problematic peers or puzzling school routines" (Hilda).

Discussion

This chapter presents a brief overview of findings from a much larger study, illustrated by one case vignette, revealing possibilities for research that can demonstrate not only whether music therapy is perceived to facilitate change but also how and why the change occurred. The findings are drawn from interpretations of evaluators who 'witnessed' music therapy practice through clinical documentation.

The music therapy practice they examined was a natural unfolding process between therapist and child with music therapists predominantly employing child-centred improvisational approaches grounded in principles of warmth, acceptance, and genuine regard (Rogers, 1961). This non-directive and relationship-based approach is built on children's strengths and interests, thus enabling their development to occur naturally within collaborative musicking (Geretsegger et al., 2015). Readers are brought close to the experiences of the evaluators who are examining music therapy practice undertaken in relevant real-world contexts (Edwards, 2002, 2005). Findings therefore have high ecological validity.

The children described in the case reports were, like other autistic children, highly motivated by music, making it an extremely useful medium for change. When children are offered favoured activities and can choose how they engage with them, they are empowered to play, explore, and make sense of their world. The predominantly broad goals employed by the clinicians and the non-directive research protocol used in this study enabled the children to develop in multiple and various ways according to their individual abilities and readiness for change. Using the benefit of hindsight, their growth across a wide variety of domains could be highlighted and valued. Their progress did not need to be judged against predefined criteria and/or against their peers. These concepts fit well with contemporary models of disability which do not judge children according to how well they adjust their behaviours to fit into a neurotypical world.

On the other hand, while evaluators who knew the children unanimously agreed that the broad goals set for the children were appropriate, two of the other experts who had backgrounds in applied behavioural analysis called for more clarity and specificity. This is important, because it suggests there is an ongoing need to promote an agenda for therapy that emphasises agency, meaningful participation, and general well-being over the achievement of specific learning and developmental tasks. Music therapists who employ a child-centred approach believe children will reach their potential when barriers are removed, and they are given a safe and supportive environment for growth (Rogers, 1961), a premise that aligns well with social and cultural models of disability (Pickard, 2019).

The findings that children progressed in diverse ways across multiple domains, also demonstrates the complexities of engaging in positivist research, which demands precise and predetermined research questions and measures. Qualitative synthesis approaches such as the one employed in this study are interpretive, and primarily concerned with generating a new interpretation or theory rather than outcomes (Pilkington, 2018). However, the qualitative concept of multiple truths allows for generation of 'a truth' in context rather than 'the truth'. It is possible to transfer knowledge extracted from rich descriptions of individual cases to another and to infer generalisability (Pilkington, 2018). In this project between seven and 11 evaluators judged each case, and cross-case analysis of the total 86 evaluations suggests that child-centred improvisational music therapy has positive outcomes for autistic children.

Acknowledgements

Dr Daphne Rickson gratefully acknowledges the IHC Foundation, and Victoria University of Wellington, New Zealand, for funding the research described in her chapter. She also gratefully acknowledges all the music therapists, children, family members, and other autism experts who were involved in the research.

References

Aigen, K. (2015). A critique of evidence-based practice in music therapy. *Music Therapy Perspectives, 33*, 12–24.

American Psychiatric Association. (2013). *Diagnostic criteria from DSM-V*. American Psychiatric Association.

Anastasiou, D., & Kauffman, J. M. (2012). Disability as cultural difference: Implications for special education. *Remedial and Special Education, 33*(3), 139–149. http://dx.doi.org/10.1177/0741932510383163

Bakan, M. B. (2018). Introduction. In M. B. Bakan (Ed.), *Speaking for ourselves: Conversations on life, music, and autism*. Oxford Scholarship Online: Oxford University Press. http://dx.doi.org/10.1093/oso/9780190855833.003.0001

Baker, L. M. (2010). Music therapy: Diversity, challenge and impact. *International Journal of Disability, Development & Education, 57*(3), 335–340. http://dx.dio.org/10.1080/1034912X.2010.501254

Baron-Cohen, S. (2017). Editorial perspective. Neurodiversity: A revolutionary concept for autism and psychiatry. *Journal of Childhood Psychology and Psychiatry, 58*, 744–747.

Bergmann, T. (2016). Music therapy for people with autism spectrum disorder. In J. Edwards (Ed.), *The Oxford handbook of music therapy*. Oxford University Press. https://doi.org/10.1093/oxfordhb/9780199639755.013.3

Bieleninik, L., Geretsegger, M., Mossler, K., Drusmus, J. A., Thompson, G., Gattino, G., Elefant, C., Gottfried, T., Igliozzi, R., Muratori, F., Suvini, F., Kim, J., Crawford, M. J., Odell Miller, H., Oldfield, A., Casey, O., Finnemann, J., Carpente, J. A., Park, A. L., Grossi, E., & Gold, C. (2017). Effects of improvisational music therapy vs enhanced standard care on symptom severity amount children with autism spectrum disorder. The TIME-A randomized clinical trial *Journal of the American Medical Association, 318*(6), 525–535. Mawhood

Borgnakke, K. (2017). Meta-ethnography and systematic reviews – linked to the evidence movement and caught in a dilemma. *Ethnography and Education: Meta-ethnographic Synthesis in Education: Challenges, Aims and Possibilities, 12*(2), 194–210. https://doi.org/10.1080/17457823.2016.1253027

Broder-Fingert, S., Feinberg, E., & Silverstein, M. (2017). Music therapy for children with autism spectrum disorder. *Journal of the American Medical Association, 318*(6), 523–524.

Campbell, C. (2008). Further towards an affirmation model. In T. Campbell, F. Fontes, L. Hemingway, A. Soorenian, & C. Till (Eds.), *Disability studies; Emerging insights and perspectives*. The Disability Press.

Carpente, J. A., & LaGasse, A. B. (2014). Music therapy for children with autism spectrum disorder. In B. Wheeler (Ed.), *Handbook of music therapy* (pp. 290–301). Guilford Press.

Carr, M. (2001). *Assessment in early childhood settings: Learning stories.* Paul Chapman.

Edwards, J. (2002). Using the evidence-based medicine framework to support music therapy post in health care settings. *British Journal of Music Therapy, 16,* 29–34.

Edwards, J. (2005). Possibilities and problems for evidence-based practice in music therapy. *The Arts in Psychotherapy, 32*(44), 293–301.

Else, B., & Wheeler, B. (2010). Music therapy practice: Relative perspectives in evidence-based reviews [Review]. *Nordic Journal of Music Therapy, 19*(1), 23. https://doi.org/10.1080/08098130903377407

Evans, B. (2018). *The autism paradox: How an autism diagnosis became both a clinical label and an identity: A stigma to be challenged and a status to be embraced.* Aeon. Retrieved November 24, 2018, from https://aeon.co/essays/the-intriguing-history-of-the-autism-diagnosis

Geretsegger, M. (2019). *Resonating research – What is needed to make music therapy research and implementation more relevant, meaningful, and innovative?* Plenary address to 11th EMTC Conference: Fields of Resonance. June 2019, Aalborg, Denmark.

Geretsegger, M., Elefant, C., Mössler, K. A., & Gold, C. (2014). Music therapy for people with autism spectrum disorder. *The Cochrane Database of Systematic Reviews, 6.* http://vuw.summon.serialssolutions.com

Geretsegger, M., Holck, U., Carpente, J. A., Elefant, C., Kim, J., & Gold, C. (2015). Common characteristics of improvisational approaches in music therapy for children with autism spectrum disorder: Developing treatment guidelines. *Journal of Music Therapy, 52*(2), 258–281.

Heaton, J. (2004). What is secondary analysis. In *Reworking qualitative data.* Sage Research Methods Online.

James, R., Sigafoos, J., Green, V., Lancioni, G., O'Reilly, M., Lang, R., Davis, T., Carnett, A., Achmadi, D., Gevarter, C., & Marschik, P. (2015, March 1). Music therapy for individuals with autism spectrum disorder: A systematic review. *Review Journal of Autism and Developmental Disorders, 2*(1), 39–54.

Janzen, T. B., & Thaut, M. H. (2018). Rethinking the role of music in the neurodevelopment of autism spectrum disorder. *Music and Science, 1,* 1–18. https://doi.org/10.1177/2059204318769639

Kapp, S. K., Gillespie-Lynch, K., Sherman, L. E., & Hutman, T. (2013, January). Deficit, difference, or both? Autism and neurodiversity. *Developmental Psychology, 49*(1), 59–71. http://dx.doi.org/10.1037/a0028353

Khundrakpam, B. S., Lewis, J. D., Kostopoulos, P., Carbonell, F., & Evans, A. (2017). Cortical thickness abnormalities in autism spectrum disorders through late childhood, adolescence, and adulthood: A large-scale MRI study. *Cerebral Cortex, 27,* 721–1731.

Kinn, L. G., Holgersen, H., Ekeland, T. J., & Davidson, L. (2013). Metasynthesis and bricolage: An artistic exercise of creating a collage of meaning. *Qualitative Health Research, 23,* 1285–1292. https://doi.org/10.1177/1049732313502127

McFerran, K., & Silverman, M. (2018). *A guide to designing research questions for beginning music therapy researchers.* American Music Therapy Association.

Ne'eman, A. (2010). The future (and the past) of autism advocacy, or why the ASA's magazine, the advocate, wouldn't publish this piece. *Disability Studies Quarterly, 30*(1). https://doi.org/10.18061/dsq.v30i1.1059

Otera, M. (2013). Is the movement of evidence-based practice a real threat to music therapy? *Voices: A World Forum for Music Therapy, 13*(2).

Pickard, B. (2019). Valuing neuro diversity: A humanistic, non-normative model of music therapy exploring Roger's person-centred approach with young adults with autism spectrum conditions. In H. Dunn, E. Coombes, E. Maclean, H. Mottram, & J. Nugent (Eds.), *Music therapy and autism across the lifespan: A spectrum of approaches* (pp. 271–296). Jessica Kingsley.

Pilkington, H. (2018). Employing meta-ethnography in the analysis of qualitative data sets on youth activism: A new tool for transnational research projects? *Qualitative Research*, *18*(1), 108–130. https://doi.org/10.1177/1468794117707805

Reschke-Hernandez, A. E. (2011, Sum). History of music therapy treatment interventions for children with autism [Article]. *Journal of Music Therapy*, *48*(2), 169–207.

Rickson, D. (2021). Family members' and other experts' perceptions of music therapy with children on the autism spectrum in New Zealand: Findings from multiple case studies. *The Arts in Psychotherapy*, 101833. https://doi.org/10/j.aip.2021.101833

Rickson, D., Castelino, A., Molyneux, C., Ridley, H., & Upjohn-Beatson, E. (2016). What evidence? Designing a mixed methods study to investigate music therapy with children who have autism spectrum disorder (ASD), in New Zealand contexts. *The Arts in Psychotherapy*, *50*, 119–125.

Rogers, C. R. (1961). *On becoming a person*. Houghton Mifflin.

Silverman, M. (2010). Integrating music therapy into the evidence-based treatments for psychiatric consumers. *Music Therapy Perspectives*, *28*, 4–10.

Slootsky, V., & Gold, C. (2016). Music therapy for autism spectrum disorder. In M. Hashefi (Ed.), *Music therapy in the management of medical conditions* (pp. 47–56). Nova Science.

Swain, J., & French, S. (2000). Towards an affirmation model of disability. *Disability & Society*, *15*(4), 569–582. https://doi.org/10.1080/09687590050058189

Waterhouse, L., London, E., & Gillberg, C. (2016, December 1). ASD validity. *Review Journal of Autism and Developmental Disorders*, *3*(4), 302–329. https://doi.org/10.1007/s40489-016-0085-x

Wheeler, B. L., & Bruscia, K. E. (Eds.). (2016). *Music therapy research* (3rd ed.). Barcelona Publishers.

Wigram, T., & Gold, C. (2006). Music therapy in the assessment and treatment of autistic spectrum disorder: Clinical application and research evidence. *Child: Care, Health and Development*, *32*(5), 535–542.

Wimpory, D., & Gwilym, E. (2019). Musical interaction therapy (MIT) for children with autistic spectrum conditions (ASCs): Underlying rationale, clinical practice and research evidence. In H. Dunn, E. Coombes, E. Maclean, H. Mottram, & J. Nugent (Eds.), *Music therapy and autism across the lifespan: A spectrum of approaches*, (pp. 97–136). Jessica Kingsley.

World Health Organisation. (2019). *Autism spectrum disorders*. World Health Organisation. Retrieved August 20, 2020, from www.who.int/news-room/fact-sheets/detail/autism-spectrum-disorders

10 In circle

The benefits of dance as a community practice

Sian Palmer

Introduction

> The circle forms.
> A gathering of peacock greens and weaver yellows
> The women's fabrics sing of their heritage.
> The rhythm sounds.
> Barefoot dancers begin to sway
> To the beat.
> The circle turns.
> Anticlockwise.
> One footstep
> At a time
> Traveling forwards:
> I have your back, you have mine.
> Backwards now:
> I trust you. It's safe here.
> And towards the centre:
> I see you, you see me.
> I am because you are.
> Thank you.
> Celebrating, being celebrated.
> A kaleidoscope of diversity.
> A circle of unity.
> We are the rhythm, the rhythm is us.
> We are the dance, the dance is us.
> We are the circle, the circle is us.

S. Palmer (2020)

African Women in Dialogue Conference in 2019 (AFWID): women's voice and power as agents of change

One thousand women from all 55 African countries gathered to explore the conference theme. I was asked to offer dance to build relationships among group members, to offer a space for personal and collective stories to be shared, and as an opportunity to debrief and process the conference content. I worked

DOI: 10.4324/9781003082897-14

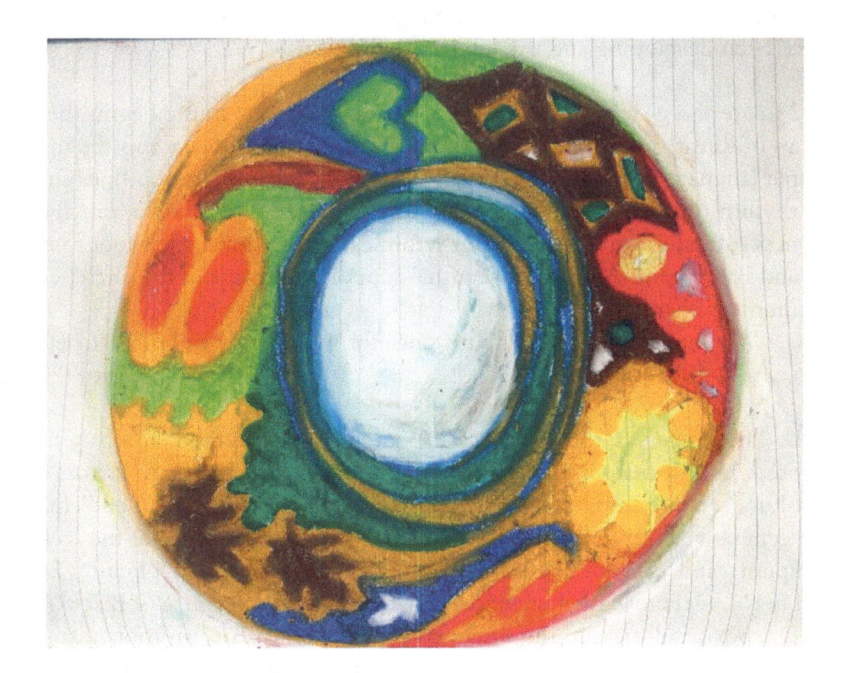

Figure 10.1 Facilitator: reflections on dance circle with AFWID group

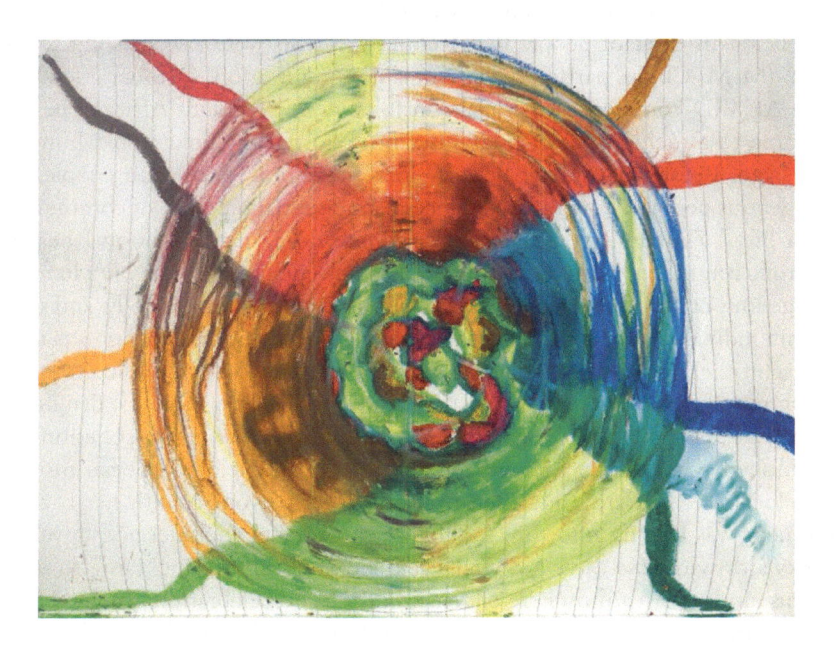

Figure 10.2 Facilitator: reflections on dance circle with AFWID group

with them using Expressive Movement (EM), a movement meditation form I have been developing and teaching since 2009.

> I invite the group to take off their shoes. When the music begins there is an outbreath; we no longer need to try to communicate across the multiple language barriers. There is an ease with which the group finds shared rhythm together. Participants naturally orientate into a circle. Initial shyness softens as we find a simple rhythmical stamp, shifting left foot to right and back again. A feeling of mutual support is present in the circle; community is here.
>
> "My humanity is bound up in yours, for we can only be human together."
>
> Desmond Tutu (2000)

Banks (2019) refers to the dance circle as a retained ancestral tradition "a time-honored African custom that has endured dismemberment due to factors such as cultural suppression, colonialism, and geographical displacement" (p. 2). The generative culture that emerges in circle dancing is a result of the feelings of support and protection that the circle structure creates (DeFrantz, 2001, pp. 11–16). DeFrantz attributes circle dancing to the emergence of Black/African Diasporic culture and the sustained connection to African roots. Dancing in circles supports connection and integration, building relationship, developing empathy, and enhancing feelings of togetherness and mutuality.

"I felt some sort of comfort and security. . . . I would say (the dance) opened me . . . it welcomed me joining with other people, and I felt so secure and safe being in front of people that I could see who were also dancing to the beat" (M. M. Chulu, participant, personal communication, October 20, 2020). The AFWID conference took place in Johannesburg, South Africa. The city is home to a melting pot of migrants who followed the gold rush a hundred years ago. Before the mining began, "Jozi" was home to the San people, the indigenous people who practised dance as an essential medium of communion with life. "The day we stop dancing, we are dead" (San traditional healer). A strong reminder of dance as an integral and essential part of daily life in many indigenous cultures, this reflects the indivisible nature of mind, body, and spirit within individual and community, with dance as a medium that connects us all to each other and to the source of life. This dance at AFWID called together a community of 23 women: activists, community leaders, mothers, daughters, sisters, and elders from all over Africa. A key moment of group cohesion was established when group members gravitated into a circle and began moving anticlockwise, forwards, and then backwards. Each woman with her back to the next was leaning into this, looking back over her shoulder and travelling backwards with ease. 'I've got your back and you've got mine' came to mind in this motion. An atmosphere of warmth, care, and celebration unfolded from there. Group members made eye contact and shared in smiles and laughter, mirroring and responding to each other's movement.

Humans have gathered in circles since we lit our first fires around 400,000 years ago if not earlier (Dibble & Sandgathe, 2017). We gathered in circles to keep ourselves and loved ones safe, to nurture our relationships. In circles we share food and soak up the warmth of the fire and conversation. We learn through the stories shared, those lived and imagined. We engage in ritual celebration and conversation through music, song, and dance. Traditionally, dance circles are held outdoors and call community members "to commemorate life occasions such as youth initiations, weddings, harvest celebrations, and more" (Banks, 2019, p. 1).

To this day, we gather in circles to engage in community practice and in group psychotherapy, to develop and enhance our intrapersonal, interpersonal, and transpersonal relationships. Schmais (1985, as cited in Fischman, 2017) dance movement therapist pioneer, speaks of the circle as a communal space where harmony can be felt in moving together. All community members stand shoulder to shoulder, taking a stance that is non-threatening, a shape that is democratic in structure. This shape enables us to see each other. We are protected within the circle and can open to one another and ourselves. In this way, we relate and form healthy attachments, attuning to and sensing the needs of one another while creating the conditions for our needs to be met.

Through the lenses of indigenous knowledge, psychology, arts psychotherapy, and neuroscience, in this chapter, we take a closer look at the positive impact that dancing together has on our brains and relationships. I use the words *movement* and *dance* interchangeably here. I encourage all people to recognise themselves as dancers, naturally able to dance.

We are the dance, the dance is us: origins of the practice

On my return to Johannesburg after completing my MA in drama and movement therapy (Sesame) in 2009, I founded a movement meditation that I call Expressive Movement (EM). This brings together groups of people and supports them in returning to the medium of spontaneous dance to enable and develop connection, communication, and creative expression. This kinaesthetic meditation form involves moving with a musical wave progression (starting slow and increasing in tempo towards a peak and then slowing down again). Through the use of music and verbal facilitation, the facilitator encourages participants to enter into embodied presence and move with what they are sensing, feeling, or imagining, developing movement with internal sensing and in relationship. Initially, time is taken to connect with oneself and one's own movement. Dancers are then encouraged to include an awareness of each other, moving at times indirectly and at times directly in relationship.

The relational aspect of this practice supports the development of a healthy sense of self and increased capacity to authentically relate with others. The sense of self arises out of social interaction (Kelly et al., 2019). The brain is engaged in both predictive processing and generative modelling that arise out of these social exchanges. The social self develops out of the experiences arising from one's body, consciousness, and being in the world. The self is

> a thinking subject, who knows that they are thinking, who can reflect, ruminate and act on the external world and is aware of their capacities for reflexivity and agency. . . . The self is the conscious awareness of the process of actively interpreting external and internal information and stimuli.
>
> (Kelly et al., p. 268)

The community phase is the third of the five phases on the Relational Cycle of EM. These five phases include developing relationships through moving in solitude, with another, in community, with the source or breath of life, and with all of life. In each EM session, dancers are encouraged to meet one another in pairs, then fours, slowly widening the circles to include larger groups and then to the whole group. From there the group draws on imagination to take participants into the wider field of connection that includes additional communities, nature, and all of life. Dancers move spontaneously both in a circle and within the circle. Through this natural return to circle dancing, we are able to move beyond words into commonly understood expressions of mutuality and support, of interdependence and a celebration of individual identity.

Honouring the social nature of movement and moving in relationship to support overall well-being, EM includes a strong focus on dancing in circles. The inclusion of the dancing circle on the EM map is inspired by the African

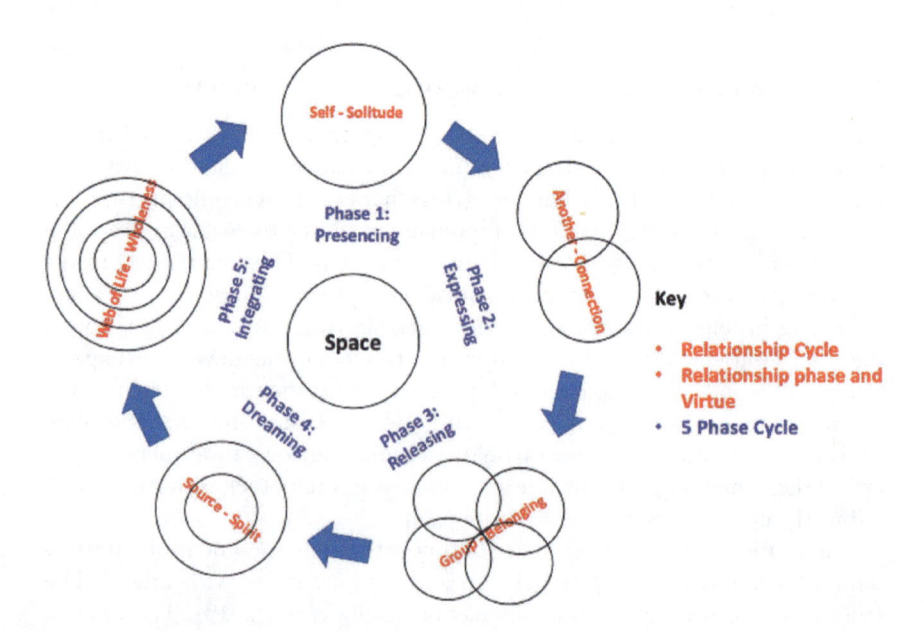

Figure 10.3 Expressive Movement map

traditional stamping circle. Marion (Billy) Lindkvist (1998), included this in the Sesame approach after travelling to South Africa, where she witnessed healing dance rituals that included drumming and stamping in a circle, as performed in the diviner's hut by the diviner's novices.

First the clappers started, and then a number of songs were sung. Various people stood up and stamped or executed one or other of the healing dance steps in a rather casual fashion. Suddenly the mood changed. The diviner took the drumsticks and introduced a different drumbeat, soon handing over the sticks to the drummer. At first the novices moved in a circle anticlockwise 'to introvert the libido' as we might say or, as the Zulus put it, "to bring the energy into the centre" (Lindkvist, 1998, p. 6).

Billy recognised the importance of stamping as an affirmation of one's existence and identity. "A man can begin to be someone when he stamps" (Lindkvist, 1998, p. 152).

Alongside my clinical training in the Sesame approach to drama and movement therapy, EM is influenced by the many dance and storytelling circles that I have been a part of from a young age, as well as my experience in ecstatic dance sessions such as 5Rhythms, founded by Gabrielle Roth (1999), and Movement Medicine, founded by Yaacov and Susannah Darling Khan (Darling Khan & Darling Khan, 2009). These all recognise our interdependence and communal nature in creative, expressive spaces, and practices. In dance we celebrate the development of our individual identity as well as look to relationships as essential to our well-being, creativity, and connection with life.

We are the rhythm, the rhythm is us: dance, rhythm, and relationship

Dance is a natural way of entering generative relationships. Lovatt (2016) highlights dance as an innate pro-social activity that promotes interpersonal communication and social bonding: "As we move together in response to music, we also move in response to each other's rhythms, helping us to form a social bond" (p. 66). Geneticists have recently found that dancers and good social communicators share two common genes:

> These researchers believe the simultaneous evolution of those genes dates back more than 1.5 million years, when group organisation and communication were essential for survival. Our prehistoric ancestors who were good dancers used those skills for bonding, social interaction, and courtship.
>
> (Mallozzi, 2020)

Together with recognising our interdependence, another of the basic principles of the EM practice, which is shared among conscious dance and movement therapy, is the understanding that we are all dancers. We have the innate ability to dance. Dancing is our birthright. Dance psychologist Peter Lovatt (2016), refers to our inherited birth rite as dancers: "Anthropologists have shown that dance-like behaviour dates back thousands of years . . . and newborn babies appear to have an innate sense of rhythm" (p. 65). At its best, this life-affirming act of dancing supports our interconnections and, as a result, enables a flow of generative communication.

The conversation that flowed after the first morning session at the AFWID conference included the spiritual, social, and political in talking about community development. Through this discussion there was an emphasis on the importance of an integrated way of being and doing which these women leaders embodied, supporting their communities in taking care of their spiritual and emotional well-being and sharing responsibility in co-creating the best possible future. Among other topics, participants brought issues of food poverty, gender-based violence, and the importance of spiritual well-being. This circle of women shared an understanding that all is embodied, everything is connected, and we live and support our living, together.

Neuroscience connections

> I see you. You see me. I am because you are.
>
> – Ubuntu philosophy

"Our human connections shape our neuronal connections throughout our lifespan" (Siegel, 1999, p. 85). Siegel's interdisciplinary framework, Interpersonal Neurobiology (INPB) or Relational Neuroscience, sees healthy living as a result of the ongoing integration of energy and information between people and within the nervous system. Siegel (2012, p. 8) refers to integration as "the organising principle that links the ways energy and information flow is shared (relationships), is shaped (the mechanisms of the embodied nervous system or, termed simply, the brain), and is regulated (the mind)." Relationship experiences change the activity and structure of the connections between our brain neurons, shaping the neuronal circuits responsible for processes such as memory, emotion, and self-awareness (Siegel 2012, p. 4). "Optimal relationships are likely to stimulate the growth of integrative fibres in the brain", thereby supporting neuronal integration and self-regulation (Siegel, 2012, p. 19). Self-regulation depends on integration in the brain and includes every aspect of regulation such as regulation of attention, emotion/affect, mood, thought, physiology, relationship, and behaviour (Siegel, 2014). INPB recognises the importance of the kind of healthy relating that dancing together cultivates.

Dancing together requires embodied presence and encourages attunement and resonance. Through attunement and empathy in this kind of relationship-oriented embodied practice, we honour difference and promote connection, supporting the inner life of oneself and each other. We practice this through feeling our body's movement and bringing our attention at the same time to each other. When dancing, we move into conversation beyond words, reflecting, supporting, and responding to one another. In good enough conditions, more intricate functions can emerge like intuition, morality, and empathy, which result in increased kindness, resilience, and health (Siegel, 2014). This practice supports the development of healthy relationships and, in turn, healthy brains. Dancing enhances the physical, emotional, mental, relational, and spiritual well-being of one another and the community.

When we breathe deeply and move spontaneously while focusing the conscious mind on our breath and movement, we get in touch with our body's internal states, developing our interoception (Christensen et al., 2018). Christensen discovered that dancers develop interoceptive accuracy which "correlates positively with measures of self-awareness and with attributes including emotional sensitivity, empathy, prosocial behavior, and efficient decision making" (p. 1).

When dancing, we feel what is going on in the body, become aware of our emotions moving within us, and bring this felt sense and our feelings into movement. Through mindful moving and embodied presence, we awaken to our imaginative and innovative minds. This way of being and creating awakens us to all our intelligences. With mind, body, and heart consciously connected, we can bring all of ourselves to meet one another in communication, co-creation, and celebration. The generative flow within us and between us enables reparative and collaborative relating. Balboa and Glacer (2019, p. 1) look at the neuroscience of conversations and the way they boost the production of hormones and neurotransmitters to create change in neural pathways and body chemistry. Key points are that communication that makes us feel good triggers increased levels of dopamine, oxytocin, and endorphins that create a sense of well-being which impacts our inner experience and state of mind. When we are in this flow, we feel safe and calm. Oxytocin is associated with love, bonding, and collaboration. When we are co-regulating in conversation, we are regulating the oxytocin and cortisol levels in each other.

Entering calm and focused presence is needed for optimal healthy relating both intra- and interpersonally. On a neurological level, we can look to Porges' (2011) polyvagal theory. Moving to a continuous rhythm in a circle regulates dancers' breathing patterns and enables them to engage in social cues such as smiling and making eye contact. These cues together with regular breathing generate a sense of calm and safety by influencing the ventral vagal network that runs from the diaphragm to the brain stem which activates the parasympathetic nervous system and regulates the body's internal rhythms (Malchiodi, 2020; Porges, 2011). Breath, rhythm, and repetition support the body's nervous system. In "activating the parasympathetic nervous system through group movement we access the neuroception of safety" (Porges, 2007, p. 13). We can connect with others through facial expression, eye contact, and body language.

Moving in circles calms the nervous system and supports interpersonal co-regulation, generating an internalised sense of well-being, relatedness and belonging among group members. With a dancing circle as a container pro-viding a sense of safety, dancers can turn towards one another and follow this non-verbal communication through movement and rhythm-making. The circle promotes the conditions for mirroring and attunement to occur while dancers make eye contact, see each other's facial expressions and gestures, and sense the inner atmospheres of one another and the atmosphere in the shared experience. Attunement is defined "as the process in which an attachment figure accurately reads an infant's nonverbal signals and responds in such a way that match the signals of the infant" (Lacson, 2019, p. 7; Wallin (2007 as cited in Lacson, 2019, p. 9). Berrol posits that "active engagement in mirroring is essential to the formation of normal attachment schema" (2006, as cited in Lacson, 2019, p. 9).

The expressive movement facilitator encourages attunement and mirroring in dancing circles through guiding participants to move with an awareness of one another and at times making the invitation to allow one's movements to be inspired or guided by a movement pattern or gesture that you see or sense in the other dancer/s. As dancers attune and mirror one another's movements, the mirror neuron system (MNS) is activated, enhancing an emotional understand-ing of the other (McGarry & Russo, 2011). Research on the MNS suggests that the brain areas responsible for perception and production of movement overlap and that these brain areas are also involved in the processing of the intention of movement (Lacson, 2019; Rizzolatti & Craighero, 2004). McGarry and Russo (2011) propose that "mirroring leads to an enhanced functioning of the MNS (in both the person mirroring and being mirrored), which leads to enhanced activation of the limbic system and thus a greater empathic response" (p. 179). IPNB recognises how we internalise the state of mind and emotional state of one another through the activation of mirror neurons and resonance circuits (Badenoch, 2008; Siegel, 1999).

Pro-social self-regulation takes place through social interaction. In a safe environment, we use gestures, facial expressions, and vocal expressions to communicate and negotiate, to maintain safety and smooth social relation-ships. According to Lapides (2011), adults have the capacity to heal their childhood attachment wounds, developing new healthy attachment patterns through attunement and mirroring non-verbal communications such as eye contact, facial expressions, and gesture. This attunement modifies the neural patterns in the right hemisphere system of the brain responsible for attach-ment, affect and self-regulation (Lacson, 2019; Schore & Schore, 2007). The neuroplasticity of the brain is influenced by attuned interpersonal relation-ships. Reparative attunement can enable rewiring of the limbic region into patterns of secure attachment (Schore, 2003). Human emotions are governed, for the most part, by the limbic system, which is a set of brain structures, including the amygdala and hippocampus, lying beneath the neocortical sur-face that covers the brain and that surrounds the thalamus at the core of the forebrain (Isaacson, 2001).

Moving together not only supports the development of empathy, but, according to Kirschner and Tomasello's (2010) study, dancing, singing, and making music together also supports the development of bonding and pro-social behaviour, which results in altruistic and collaborative actions. This may be because these activities encourage the participants "to keep a constant audiovisual representation of the collective intention and shared goal of vocalising and moving together in time – thereby effectively satisfying the intrinsic human desire to share emotions, experiences and activities with others" (p. 354).

Tarr et al. (2015, p. 3) discovered through their research that both synchrony (performing the same movement together) and exertion during dance raises our pain threshold and encourages social bonding. The release of endorphins while dancing is related to the physical exercise as well as the social element. The endogenous opioid system and, more specifically, the release of endorphins may be an important link between interpersonal synchrony and social bonding as the release of neurohormones "causes some form of social 'high', which increases positivity towards those in the vicinity" (p. 3).

Poikonen (2017) attributes the rise of rich cultures and communities to the presence of music and dancing as they promote and enhance social interaction. She speaks of dance naturally combining the basic elements of humanity being creative expression, fine-tuned and whole-body movement, touch, and collaboration. She also makes the link between dancing and the flow state, a phenomenon well researched by Csikszentmihalyi (2004), where a person is in a state of immersion and heightened focus. The flow state is connected to reduced activation of the neural network generating a relaxed state of mind together with increased feelings of contentment:

> When dancers are moving together their brains become attuned to the same frequency, their low-theta brainwaves synchronising. Brain synchronisation enables seamless cooperation and is necessary for creating both harmonic music and movement. The ability to become attuned to another person's brain frequency is essential for the function of any empathetic community.
>
> (Poikonen, 2017, pp. 3–4)

Evaluative process

In order to monitor reactions and group mood and behaviour changes before, during, and after the expressive movement session, I followed Schon's (1983) model of reflective practice. To evaluate the effectiveness of the session I held in mind four criteria: body language, eye contact, verbal communication, and the mood or atmosphere in the room. At the start of the session, I noticed that some group members came in alone and sat down on chairs, looking at their phones or crossing their arms and resting in silence. There were murmurs of conversation between some group members, and it appeared that there was some nervousness and difficulty in communicating across language barriers. Some eye contact was made between group members and with me. There was a sense of anticipation, nervousness, and resistance before we began as there can be in a group that is meeting each other for the first time. During the course of the session and afterwards, I noticed a marked shift. There was an ease in body language as the women stood together, shoulders open, arms uncrossed, openly chatting. Eye contact seemed easier to make, and there was laughter and chatter in the room, creating a warm atmosphere of cohesion. Reflecting on these changes it appeared that the dance assisted group members to feel at ease, connected, and energised.

Towards the end of 2020, I had informal contact with some members of the group, asking them what had stayed with them from our time together. The predominant theme that emerged through all conversation was the theme of togetherness and sharing that the dance supported. This was a big theme threading throughout the conference, one of mutual support and strength in solidarity. Perhaps this experience of being together, as Siegel (2014) suggests, positively shapes our neuronal connections, increasing our resilience and over-all wellbeing.

To carry out research in this area I would use a participatory action research (PAR) model. PAR is an approach used "for improving conditions and prac-tices in a range of healthcare environments, improving practitioners' own prac-tice through systematic inquiries of action, evaluation and critical reflection, the outcomes of which then inform further practice" (Koshy et al., 2010, p. 1). Regular feedback from participants as well as observations made by the facilita-tor/therapist, leads to improved practice through changes that are implemented as a result in each following stage of the research. Koshy et al. (2010) provide models for PAR.

We are the circle, the circle is us: embodying community through dancing online during the COVID-19 pandemic

"Pandemic lockdowns might be pervasive, but not all our movements are restricted. This has led to a rise in dance, as people seek fitness, stress relief, healing and connection. Live classes on Instagram and YouTube have prolifer-ated" (Mallozzi, 2020, p. 1).

During the COVID-19 pandemic, I have witnessed and experienced fear, uncertainty, and isolation. I have danced in and held online classes and seen and sensed how dancing offers both remedy and prevention. Dance calms our nervous systems, uplifts our spirits, and maintains our connections with one another. In working online with dancers practising on their own at home, I recognise the importance of creating the necessary conditions and facilitating in ways that support connection. Many have been feeling lonely and isolated because of the lockdown, missing physical touch and the feeling of dancing together in community. "More than ever, we need to dance with purpose to remind the world that humanity still exists", says Gregory Vuyani Maqoma, an acclaimed dancer and educator from South Africa, in a statement for the World Dance Alliance, Maqoma (2020).

> Our purpose is one that strives to change the world one step at a time.
> (Mallozzi, 2020)

In working online, I have come to realise that community movement does not need to take place exclusively in the physical presence of one another. We can widen these dancing circles across the globe through online practice. We can look to dance to connect us with our common humanity, unique creativity, and our capacity to co-create the best possible future. Through dancing online, using platforms such as Zoom, we widen the circles across time zones and physical borders and can celebrate our diversity and oneness. I have witnessed moments of deep resonance and generativity between and among dancers, hand gestures of giving and taking, mirroring movements that speak of seeing and being seen, dancers moving with feeling and feeling supported. I have felt and seen repetitions and ripples of rhythm and patterns of movement in the whole group, each on their own dance floor at home connected on the virtual dance floor.

I have found myself facilitating imagined circles in order to maintain the strength of this organic nature of dance and connection. Working on Zoom has its challenges. The two-dimensional nature of the screen can be alienating and render individuals feeling watched, estranged, or disconnected (Morris, 2020). In response, I decided to bring in the dancing circle through guided imaginative and embodied meditation, inviting group members to imagine someone in the Zoom session coming to stand on either side of them, someone to stand across the way from them, on the other side of the circle. Bringing in specific individuals as anchors and then imagining a whole circle moving with us creates a deep, supportive experience for the group. Group members have reflected back that they felt deeply connected to themselves, to one another and to their families, and even to their ancestors. Imagining and embodying moving in circle appears to access our orientation towards safety, connection, and collaboration, creating a feeling of wholeness, interdependence, and well-being, connecting through relational neuroscience.

Conclusion

A kaleidoscope of diversity, a circle of unity

> You know how we were all from different backgrounds and different personalities, there were old people, and there were young people, from all walks of life. Your dance class made us forget who we were. . . . It didn't matter what age. . . . After the dance we all became intertwined. We laughed, we danced, we discovered more conversation than we could speak. So dance just opened up a new perspective on how we should understand

people. . . . It helped us break the walls down and build bridges. We discovered a lot of friends because of (this dance).

(M.M. Chulu, participant, personal communication, October 20, 2020)

This reflection from an AFWID participant affirms the nature of dance as restorative and generative, supporting individual expression and group collaboration. Dancing together at AFWID initiated connection and communication beyond words, which felt important for such a multilingual, multi-ethnic group. The experience of cohesion and shared feeling of joy was tangible.

Moving in circles enables us to see one another, reflect and respond to each other, express ourselves, and create and collaborate resulting in the emergence of dynamic, supportive, and generative movement patterns that can be understood as conversations taking place beyond words. The movement patterns are at times full of joy and play, at times an expression of grief and at times simple, calming rhythmic motions. All aspects of life can be danced and felt and shared and responded to together. I encourage practitioners to continue facilitating dancing together in circles (physical or imagined). Keep it simple. Choose a song you like that has a steady beat and preferably one that includes some indigenous instruments. Encourage participants to gather in circle or imagine a circle gathering, to stamp their feet on the ground in rhythmic repetition, and to allow themselves to dance, to express themselves, and to feel the collective rhythm supporting them. Building bridges, crossing divides, supporting each other, and recognising our shared responsibility is paramount to co-creating the best possible present and future. Dancing can offer both remedy and prevention in this time where we need good mental health, resilience, and relationships.

Acknowledgements

I would like to thank Bunie M. Matlanyane Sexwale – my wise elder, colleague, and dear friend who invited me to present Expressive Movement at the AFWID conference.

Huge gratitude to all the women who danced!

References

Badenoch, B. (2008). *Being a brain-wise therapist: A practical guide to interpersonal neurobiology.* W. W. Norton.

Balboa, N., & Glacer, R. D. (2019). The neuroscience of conversations. *Psychology Today.* www.psychologytoday.com/gb/blog/conversational-intelligence/201905/the-neuroscience-conversations

Banks, O. C. (2019). Fare Ra Lankhi. *Journal of Dance Education,* 1–9.

Christensen, J. F. Gaigg, S. B., & Calvo-Merino, B. (2018). I can feel my heartbeat: Dancers have increased interoceptive accuracy. *Psychophysiology, 55*(4).

Csikszentmihalyi, M. (2004). Flow, the secret of happiness. *Ted.* www.ted.com/talks/mihaly_csikszentmihalyi_flow_the_secret_to_happiness

Darling Khan, Y., & Darling Khan, S. (2009). *Movement medicine: How to awaken, dance and live your dreams*. Hay House.

DeFrantz, T. F. (2001). Black bodies dancing black culture: Black Atlantic transformations. Foreword in *Embodying Liberation: The Black Body in American Dance* (pp. 11–16). LIT Verlag.

Dibble, H., & Sandgathe, D. (2017). Who started the first fire? *Sapiens*. www.sapiens.org/archaeology/neanderthal-fire/

Fischman, D. I. (2017). Understanding group shaping: Transcontextual metapatterns in body, movement and dance. *Psychotherapy: An International Journal for Theory, Research and Practice*, *12*(2), 83–97. https://doi.org/10.1080/17432979.2016.1218933

Isaacson, R. L. (2001). The limbic system. In *International Encyclopedia of the Social & Behavioral Sciences* (pp. 8858–8862). www.sciencedirect.com/topics/neuroscience/limbic-system

Kelly, M. P., Kriznik, N. M, Kinmonth, A. L., & Fletcher, P. C. (2019). The brain, self and society: A social-neuroscience model of predictive processing. *The Journal of Social Neuroscience*, *14*(3), 266–276.

Kirschner, S., & Tomasello, M. (2010). Joint music making promotes prosocial behavior in 4-year-old children. *Evolution and Human Behavior, 31*, 354–364.

Koshy, E., Koshy, V., & Waterman, H. (2010). *What is action research?* Sage. www.sagepub.com/upm-data/36584_01_Koshy_et_al_Ch_01.pdf

Lacson, F. C. (2019). Embodied attunement: A dance/movement therapy approach to working with couples. *Body, Movement and Dance in Psychotherapy*, *15*(1), 4–19. https://doi.org/10.1080/17432979.2019.1699859

Lapides, F. (2011). The implicit realm in couple therapy: Improving right hemisphere affect-regulating capabilities. *Clinical Social Work Journal*, *39*(2), 161–169.

Lindkvist, M. (1998). *Bring white beads when calling on the healer*. Rivendell House.

Lovatt, P. (2016, December). This is why we dance: *Psychology Magazine*. BBC Science Focus, 62–67.

Malchiodi, C. (2020). Tapping the healing rhythms of the vagal nerve: Self-regulation is found through the sound of your internal beat. *Psychology Today*. www.psychologytoday.com/us/blog/arts-and-health/202004/tapping-the-healing-rhythms-the-vagal-nerve

Mallozzi, M. (2020). Virtual dance parties are popular: What's behind their rise? *National Geographic*. www.nationalgeographic.com/travel/2020/04/how-dance-connects-people-during-coronavirus/

Maqoma, G. V. (2020, April, 29th). *Message for international dance day 2020*. www.iti-worldwide.org.

McGarry, L. M., & Russo, F. A. (2011). Mirroring in dance/movement therapy: Potential mechanisms behind empathy enhancement. *The Arts in Psychotherapy*, *38*(3), 178–184.

Morris, B. (2020). Why does zoom exhaust you? Science has an answer. *The Wall Street Journal*. www.wsj.com/articles/why-does-zoom-exhaust-you-science-has-an-answer-11590600269

Palmer, S. (2020). *Circle poem* (unpublished).

Poikonen, H. (2017). A dancer's brain develops in a unique way. *University of Helsinki*. www.helsinki.fi/en/news/health/a-dancers-brain-develops-in-a-unique-way

Porges, S. W. (2007). The polyvagal perspective. *Biological Psychology, 74*, 116–143. https://doi.org/10.1016/j.biopsycho.2006.06.009

Porges, S. W. (2011). *The polyvagal theory*. W. W. Norton.

Rizzolatti, G., & Craighero, L. (2004). The mirror-neuron system. *Annual Reviews of Neuroscience*, *27*, 169–192. www.scirp.org/reference/ReferencesPapers.aspx?ReferenceID=1357129

Roth, G. (1999). *Sweat your prayers: Movement as spiritual practice*. Gill Books.

Schon, D. A. (1983). *The reflective practitioner: How professionals think in action*. Basic Books.

Schore, A. (2003). *Affect regulation and the repair of the self.* W. W. Norton.

Schore, J. R., & Schore, A. N. (2007). Modern attachment theory: The central role of affect regulation in development and treatment. *Clinical Social Work Journal, 36*(1), 9–20.

Siegel, D. J. (1999). *The developing mind: Toward a neurobiology of interpersonal experience.* Guilford Press.

Siegel, D. J. (2012). Mind, brain and relationships: The interpersonal neurobiology perspective. In *The developing mind: How relationships and the brain interact to shape who we are* (2nd ed.). Guilford Press.

Siegel, D. J. (2014). Interpersonal connection, self-awareness and well-being: The art and science of integration in the promotion of health. *Stanford Medicine, X.* www.youtube.com/watch?v=bP9bT6xfhNE

Tarr, B., Launay, J., Cohen, E., & Dunbar, R. (2015). Synchrony and exertion during dance independently raise pain threshold and encourage social bonding. *Biology Letters, 11*, 20150767. https://dx.doi.org/10.1098/rsbl.2015.0767

Tutu, D. (2000). *No future without forgiveness.* Rider.

11 Mind and movement

Using the universality of neuroscience in dance movement therapy

Verity Danbold

> Dance movement therapy is the relational and therapeutic use of dance and move-
> ment to further the physical, emotional, cognitive, social, and cultural functioning
> of a person. Dance movement therapy is based on the empirically-supported unity
> of body and mind.
>
> (Dance Therapy Association of Australasia, 2017)

Globally, we are confronting a human rights crisis in mental health (Funk et al., 2013–2020, p. 1). Impacts of inadequate mental health provision are far-reaching, from the microscopic altering of individuals' DNA to the systemic impacts on national health systems. It is imperative that we respond to this crisis. Internationally, dance movement therapy (DMT) has emerged as an effective therapeutic intervention, addressing the need for client-led, culturally adaptable, and resource-light mental health support (Capello, 2016; Danbold, 2017). Increasingly, DMT is informed and validated by our expanding understanding of neuroscience. By basing interventions in what we have in common (the brain, the parasympathetic nervous system, breath), instead of what has traditionally divided us (the concept of self, the therapeutic hierarchy of client and therapist, or the misogyny of early psychotherapeutic principles), DMT can continue to work effectively within this global emergency. This will be explored through three DMT interventions targeting the brain and nervous system: mirroring, the felt sense, and grounding.

DMT recognises the universality of movement. In its most primal form, movement and connection through movement define life:

> Rhythmic input from muscles and voice, after gradually suffusing through the entire nervous system, may provoke echoes of the fetal condition when a major and perhaps principal external stimulus to the developing brain was the mother's heartbeat.
>
> (McNeil, 2009, p. 7)

From the first moment of conception, we move. Footage of in vitro fertilised embryos show the quivering, microscopic cells splitting and dividing. This

DOI: 10.4324/9781003082897-15

blastocyst will tumble down in the uterus, embedding itself into the uterine walls, which themselves might cramp and twinge at the intrusion, the first kinaesthetic link between mother and child. The earliest links of movement and body are visible on an ultrasound; the embryo's heart will beat an uneven rhythm until the brain is developed enough to control its parts. Kestenberg Movement work can begin antenatally as

> attunement, through sharing muscle tension rhythms, produces feelings of mutuality and responsiveness to needs and feelings, as expressed through muscular tension-flow. The process of kinesthetic attunement required for fetal movement notation contributes to the foundation for attachment between mother and unborn child.
>
> (Loman, 2016, p. 226)

As this baby grows, the brain will continue to guide the multitude of movements that make up life. Whilst reading, your eyes dart on this page, your breath rises and falls, perhaps your stomach gurgles and squeezes. It will continue to do so until death, which could well be defined as the final absence of movement. This march from conception to death is universal, embedding movement-based interventions in our most primal markers of human existence.

Movement not only defines our individual existence but our global evolution as well. Since prehistoric times, humans have recognised dance and movement as tools for growth and recovery (Garfinkel, 2011, p. 206). Prehistoric cave drawings emphasise the role of dance in prehistoric civilisations, their images of dance not dissimilar to some contemporary dancers and dance therapists' own dance notations. Garfinkel draws on McNeil's (2020) theory that dance and evolution are linked. There is merit in their theory: dance 'maps' helped indigenous communities to remember fertile hunting grounds; courting dances helped identify the strongest and most able partners; undulating hip dances encouraged mothers to prepare for safer births or helped communities process trauma that might otherwise have led to epigenetic alterations. If we work from this theory, that dance and movement quite literally shaped our contemporary brains, it is only fitting that we now return to dance and movement to explore its inner workings.

The pioneers of DMT, such as Chace (cited in Tosey, 1992, p. 254) and Payne (1992) similarly called on dance's capacity to connect and heal, grounding themselves in the same principles of mirrored movement, embodiment, and rhythm. Over time, dance movement therapists formalised, in practice and academia, what had been 'known' to humanity since prehistoric times. By combining this with more contemporary understanding and theory of therapy and mental health, DMTs moved dance from therapeutic to therapy, a change marked in practice, process, and outcome. It is now defined as "a relational process in which client/s and therapist engage in an empathic creative process using body movement and dance to assist integration of emotional, cognitive, physical, social and spiritual aspects of self" (Association for Dance Movement

Psychotherapy, UK, 2020). Here it is important to note that 'dance' movement therapy can sometimes be a misnomer as many DMT clients choose not to dance. Instead, we draw on the understanding that we are constantly moving: breath, heartbeat, fine twitch movement, as examples. Even in the moment a client says they do not dance, their brain is firing off a multitude of signals promoting movements, which form the words, to perhaps shift uncomfortably in their chair or sustain eye contact. Our improved understanding about how the brain/mind/body link creates human experience is reflected in our therapeutic practice. From improved understanding of the trauma response to understanding how brain chemistry impacts addiction, the profession continues to value research and to invest in opportunities which expand and extend the field.

Therapy, as a provision and a profession, has too often been the privilege of a wealthy, predominately white minority, yet, globally, an estimated 792 million people or one in 10 people, have a mental health condition (York, 2020; World Health Organisation [WHO], 2019). Women and girls are disproportionately impacted (WHO, 2019). Nearly two thirds of this population will not access professional mental health support. There is a global need for therapeutic interventions. While the World Health Organization's (WHO's) Mental Health Action Plan (2013–2020) recognises a commitment to mental health provision as central to achieving overarching health goals, it is clear that both provision and uptake of such provision are lacking. On average, countries invest less than 2% of their annual budget in mental health, revealing the systemic extent of the problem (WHO, 2019). While government investment and provision doubtlessly stand as a barrier to good mental health, communities themselves must work to fight the stigma of mental health to improve uptake of those services provided. The Psychological Health and Wellness Clinic, a therapy organisation based in Dhaka, Bangladesh, recently reported that only 8% of adults living in the country would seek mental health assistance if needed (PHWC website, 2021). Human Rights Watch reported hundreds of people living with mental health conditions are shackled in more than 60 countries (Sharma, 2020). Reflecting on acceptance of mental health support in Latin and South America, Alarcon (2003) writes:

> This is aggravated by deeply rooted cultural characteristics, particularly those related to shame and guilt in the perception of cases of mental illness among families, distorted help-seeking patterns, religious and folk beliefs about causes and treatment, and the sheer unavailability of appropriate mental health services.
>
> (p. 54)

We must reflect, as practitioners and providers, on how our mental health provision responds to a global crisis. Much of therapeutic practice, both verbal and creative, was founded and formalised in research and beliefs that reflected the Eurocentric prejudices and biases of its time. This adds a further barrier to uptake of mental health services demonstrating the need for therapists to reflect on their own cultural bias within their training and practice. Recent backlash against Laban Movement Analysis, in its historical context of racism and anti-Semitism, indicates a need for DMTs to question the underlying theoretical and philosophical basis of their practice (Dickson, 2016, p. 7). If we take a concept like 'timeliness', which to clients in the Global North (formerly referred to as 'the developed world') may create a sense of boundaries, respect, and form, to their counterparts in the Global South (formerly 'the third' or 'developing world') may bring echoes of neo-colonialism, othering, and privilege. Based in Kolkata, the DMT non-governmental organisation (NGO) Kolkata Sanved's Sampoornata model (Chakraborty, 2004) explicitly states 'empowerment and human rights' as therapy aims, recognising that these may not be a given in certain communities. Kolkata Sanved frequently employs former clients, challenging the practice of Western therapy, as new clients see themselves actively reflected in their dance movement therapists and practitioners. Even the creative expression so highly prized by creative arts therapists may be alien in communities where years of rote learning have systemically diminished space for creativity. Reflecting on the Western epistemology of rationalism, Kinouani (2017, para. 14) challenges the widely utilised cognitive behaviour therapy approach, noting that

> [i]t is one thing to encourage people to seek 'objective evidence' to help disprove the belief that everyone hates them but, quite another to ask people of colour to back up their belief that they are experiencing racism. Direct objective evidence of racism is rarely available. And it is precisely because of difficulties in 'objectively' evidencing oppression that people living in racialised and in other bodies marked as Other, have had to develop ways to apprehend reality that are not dependent upon rationalism. . . . In this context, invalidating our ways of knowing and navigating the world is not only likely psychologically harmful; it is also a social act which serves to negate racism and therefore reproduces white supremacy.

While responsibility lies both with governments, NGOs/international organisations and communities to provide adequate mental health care funding, the responsibility for providing culturally aware therapy lies with the therapist. It is not a responsibility from which to shirk. Drawing on neuroscience moves away from culturally biased theories to something more universal: the human brain and nervous system.

DMT addresses some of the barriers to accessing therapy globally. Non-verbal DMT is practiced in situations in which there may be no shared language or with limited, non- or pre-verbal clients. DMT is client-led, enabling clients to draw on their familiar socio-cultural uses of dance and movement. While the extent to which props are used varies considerably, there is scope for DMT to be conducted entirely through the body, ideal for resource-poor settings. In working through movement, DMT can look and feel vastly different from the stereotypical view of the Freudian couch. For some, this can help reduce the fear and stigma of therapy. The act of reclaiming the body through movement is both powerful and political, an important step in a global climate of misogyny, gender-based violence, trans- and homophobia, racism, and torture. While the mind–body link has been divorced in the global North, a heavy stigmatism attached to the concept of psychosomatic illness; elsewhere, the mind and body remain strongly tied. Working within a form that addresses the profound link between mind and body acknowledges a client's own understanding of their experience.

DMT has been both legitimised and improved by advances in neuroscience. Perhaps most profound is the increased recognition that experiences are stored in the body (Loman & Foley, 1996). While therapists see this in the macro-expression of the human body or the movement of groups, scientists are increasingly seeing evidence of trauma 'stored' in the body – in the division of DNA, the flow of cortisol to the fetus, and even the increased prevalence of female live births in areas of systemic trauma events (Youssef et al., 2018; Song, 2009). The seminal (1995–1997) Adverse Childhood Experience study (Felitti et al., 1998) revealed the extent to which adverse childhood experiences impact mental and physical health as adults, noting that the health of millions of Americans might have been improved by the prevention of these experiences. A mother's own unresolved trauma may inhibit her brain's reaction to her infant's distress, creating an attachment trauma cycle which not only impacts the child's mental well-being but may also prevent the mother from responding to cues of hunger, pain, or tiredness which further adversely affects the child's development (Kim et al., 2014). Not all evidence lies in adverse experiences, the work of Kestenberg and Anna Freud reflect an improved understanding of infant and early childhood brain and body development, the suckling, rolling, mimicking milestones of growth that can be seen worldwide.

Mirroring

The intersection of neuroscience and DMT can be observed in mirroring using the felt sense (Gendlin, 1981) to understand trauma response and grounding. Mirroring, as a form of kinaesthetic understanding, is present in our everyday lives, making it a familiar form of communication for clients. Perhaps the most well-known marker of mirroring in everyday life is the ever-contagious yawn. It is possible that even reading *yawn* may have triggered a response in the reader (Gupta & Mittal, 2013). Talking to a loved one, we naturally slip into moments of mirroring, such as adopting a similar stance, tone, or inflection. In a more sophisticated use of mirroring, a wailing baby may be comforted by their carer who, at first, mirrors and demonstrates empathy with their child's heightened state by exclamations and a fretful expression and gradually utilises contrasting mirroring of a calm and reassuring tone to assure the baby their needs will be met. With the increased move towards an online world, people conversing in different time zones may begin to mirror the circadian markers of their counterpart, demonstrating both the innate human drive to mirror, and a potential challenge to online working as our bodies lose grounding in their own 'real-life' natural cues.

In the brain, mirror neurons form the basis of our mirroring response. While there are a variety of theories about the evolutionary role of mirror neurons, including their role in speech development, it is their role in the capacity for empathy that plays most strongly in a therapeutic relationship. Mirror neurons fire even when the stimulus is not acting on the individual body. The reader is invited to imagine witnessing someone cutting themselves while chopping vegetables or seeing someone trip up a flight of stairs in front of a large crowd. Note the response in your own body. Perhaps there was a wince or a slight dizziness at the cut or a flush of embarrassment at the thought of falling up the stairs. All these responses are the result of mirror neurons. By provoking a physical/emotional response in our body, mirror neurons allow us to 'read' others outside ourselves. For dance movement therapists, this forms an important aspect of embodiment "the bodily phenomena in which the body as a living organism, body movement and person-environment interaction play central roles in the explanation of perception, cognition, affect, attitudes, behaviour and their interpretation" (Koch & Fischman, 2011, p. 4).

One in 160 children worldwide is on the autism spectrum many of whom are undiagnosed and have limited access to support (WHO, 2019). Increased reporting, expansion of diagnostic criteria, and better diagnosis reporting, all suggest this proportion may well continue to rise. While it is accepted that there is no cure, effective therapeutic intervention can support people on the autism spectrum and their families. The WHO recognises the importance of this as a worldwide responsibility. Dance therapy has been increasingly widely recognised as a therapeutic intervention for autism spectrum disorder (ASD). As Mastrominico (2018, para. 10) notes,

> [g]iven the potential of sensory and motor challenges to impact individuals' availability to engage socially, the facilitation of multiple ways of connecting to sensory and motor experiences including moving in and out of interpersonal synchrony within the context of an interaction in DMT, may contribute to its therapeutic success in treating individuals with ASD.

The causes of ASD remain contested. One potential theory, the 'broken mirror' theory, stems from Iacobini's 2006 study, which demonstrated that "fMRI [functional magnetic resonance imaging] data show that children with ASD have reduced Mirror Neuron System (MNS) activity during social mirroring and that MNS activity correlates with the severity of disease: the higher the impairment, the lower the MNS activity in ASD" (Iacoboni & Depratto, 2006, p. 8). This led to the theory that individuals with ASD have impaired MNS resulting in delayed or non-existent language development, the perceived lack of empathy, and the inability to read and respond to social cues. However, the research of Schulte-Rüther et al. (2016, p. 298) contradicts the 'broken mirror' theory noting that the mirror mechanism for automatic facial emotions remain intact, "but is not associated with complex social cognitive abilities such as emotion understanding and empathy." Whether working to nurture the growth of a functioning MNS or working to counter the impacts of its impairment, both schools of thought can lead their subscribers to the same conclusion: working therapeutically with MNS can be a valuable intervention.

The use of mirroring is one of DMT's earliest approaches. It can be as simple as copying the movements of another person but can be expanded to variations such as multimodal mirroring (the use of props or sounds), contrasting mirroring (moving in opposition to the primary movers, e.g. fast to their slow), or variations (working on the theme of mirroring). Body-based, it crosses both non-verbal and language barriers. Recognising the role of MNS in learning, the mirroring and sharing of movements support both fine and gross motor skills development. Yet mirroring is more than simply replicating movement. For many therapists, mirroring is better understood as its therapeutic synonym: kinetic empathy.

Mirroring is a complex form of interacting that involves more than the imitation of the external form of the movement. Great attention is paid to the empathetic reflection of the affective state of the patient in movement. "The intentions of the patient are reflected back to them through the process of picking up their intentional themes and structuring these in subsequent movement sequences" (Eberhard-Kaechele, 2012, p. 283).

In DMT, the 'mirror-er' empathetically reflects the mover's emotional state back to them, helping to structure, illuminate and communicate themes within this body dialogue. For a client with ASD, for example, this transition from mechanically copying movements to mirroring and responding in tone is an important process in therapy and a vital step towards improving their interpersonal relationships in the outside world.

Using the felt sense to understand trauma response

Trauma is a universal experience and one of the most enduring themes of human existence that has shaped the lives and brains of humans since time immemorial. Early childhood trauma shapes the brain, irreparably damaging it, as revealed in the magnetic resonance imaging (MRI) research scans of Wittbrodt et al. (2019). For many who experience trauma, the event may be followed by an ongoing period of dysregulation, the symptoms of which may be clinically grouped as post-traumatic stress disorder (PTSD)/cPTSD (complex PTSD). Furthermore, the neurological response to trauma results in a reduced capacity to engage in new learning or to accurately create and store memory. This inability to store memory is an important survival mechanism, but conversely may be distressing for trauma survivors.

The trauma response, sometimes referred to as 'flight, fight, freeze', is one of the best advocates for the use of DMT as a treatment modality. Trauma is perceived first in the primitive brain, releasing a flood of chemicals effectively shutting off the more cognitive part of the brain, and focusing on the body responses of fight, flight, or freeze. This results in the brain storing trauma as a pre-verbal event. As a result, verbal/cognitive therapies may support the client to develop cognitive coping strategies but do not address the somatic response to trauma where the body memories are stored. Working through body-based therapies enable a client to process, rather than manage, the trauma (Ogden & Minton, 2000, p. 150).

DMT often uses the felt sense. Gendlin (1981, p. 35) writes, "A felt sense is an odd sort of datum, a holistic sense of what is unresolved, a sense of the whole thing . . . the felt sense is perhaps the deepest kind of 'letting form'." He further described it as 'a special kind of internal bodily awareness, a body sense of meaning'. This can strike clients as too abstract a concept, something too esoterically 'therapy' to be of value in the real world. We can describe it as 'a gut feeling' or 'tummy talking'. However, it is perhaps best understood experientially, worked first as concrete practical examples before moving to the use of movement metaphors that underpin DMT. The reader is now invited to try the following 'felt sense' exercise for themselves, first reading the following paragraph and subsequently closing their eyes and recalling its instructions.

> *You are, at this very moment, in contact with the ground or a chair. It may be that you are standing or sitting on a hard-backed chair or reclining on a sofa. It may be a hot day and your bare skin comes into contact with the surface, that you are in uncomfortable shoes, or you are reading this on the bus in a warm winter coat. Whatever your circumstances, take a moment to note all the concrete observations that you feel: Are the pillows hard or soft? Is the carpet woven or thick pile? Make note of as many of these concrete observations as you can. With time, you can begin to affix sensations and thought to them. Does the seat comfortably hold you, or are you tensing your muscles? Are the tiles beneath your feet cooling or cold? What memories or associations come from this seat? Take a moment to reflect on how your body senses and reacts to something as simple as your seat.*

A therapist may use the exercise above in supporting a client to reflect on the felt sense within a therapeutically safe context, such as their response to sitting. By raising a client's awareness of the felt sense, these same principles can then be applied to in-depth client work. For example, how is the felt sense experienced when discussing an argument with a partner, responding to a therapist's question or when recalling a traumatic event? The therapist might draw on their own felt sense to support their understanding and interpretation of client material. Perhaps, in noting their own physical sensations, the therapist might verbalise something that felt stuck bodily for the client. In group work, using the felt sense can give rise to shared themes and experiences, supporting clients to feel less alone in their experiences or to give word and form to something intangible.

Trauma work may initially begin as psychoeducation, encouraging clients to understand the neurobiological reasons behind their thoughts and actions.

Clients may experience a range of responses to trauma, from insomnia to uncontrolled rage, all of which can be tied back to the dysregulated amygdala. Psycho-education can address questions such as why a client could not fight back or why a certain smell can, years later, produce such a visceral response of panic. In theory, imparting this information can provide a robust retort to the uncertainty and shame trauma provokes. In practice, there are barriers to approaching this from a psycho-educative angle. Symptoms of trauma can feel so resolutely physical, such as the overwhelming breathlessness and pounding heart of a panic attack, that placing the onus on the brain seems far-fetched. As discussed earlier, the term *psychosomatic* has become stigmatised in the global North. The brain, for many clients, remains a mystery. Educational provisions in few countries are of a standard that neuroscience will be regularly taught, and this is assuming access to education, with one in five children out of education globally (UNESCO, 2018). There may be socio-cultural responses with explanations centring on evolution's role in our trauma response not accepted. Even when the concepts are firmly grasped as theory, it is sometimes an ongoing challenge for a client to apply them to their own lived experience.

Here is where working through the felt sense comes into its own. In defining the trauma response through abrupt actions, 'flight, fight, freeze' we acknowledge that it is a bodily process, experienced through action or lack thereof. Unresolved trauma may become held between the experiencing/reacting amygdala and the cognitive/processing frontal cortex. When exploring this in therapy, clients may use the felt sense to access the non-verbal space in which trauma is held. They may be able to move this body memory within a non-verbal reflection and movement process, developing transitory reactive movements into a movement pattern. In this process, the bodily-held trauma moves outwardly to the cognitive brain where it can be processed and safely held. The felt sense allows for the client to experience the mysterious workings of the brain bodily and to apply experiential understanding to the science. Ogden and Minton (2000, p. 158) and Siegel's (1999) Window of Tolerance (WOT) illustrates our brain existing in one of three states: hypo-arousal, hyper-arousal, and the ideal WOT. Within our window of tolerance, we feel a sense of ownership over our thoughts, feelings, and emotions, secure in our ability to respond effectively to situations, to learn and connect with others. The dysregulated brain may leave its WOT following trauma. This experience may be overwhelming physically, with increased heart rate, dizziness, or marked by an 'out of body' sense, such as in dissociation. Working with the felt sense, clients can identify these responses and strengthen their individualised concept of what it means to be within their WOT. It can further support clients to develop individual strategies to remain within their window of tolerance. They may develop the capacity to recognise the more subtle signs of dysregulation, enabling them to put strategies in place sooner.

Grounding

One challenge to therapy in the Global South, and increasingly worldwide, is the lack of resources for long-term therapy. This may be paired with the conviction that therapy can be too exposing in situations in which the possibility for re-traumatisation exists. Unfortunately, for the millions of displaced people, those who remain in conflict zones, or those trapped in abusive marriages, this may mean a lifetime of denied access to mental health support. The development of short-term interventions is therefore vital.

Porges' (1994) polyvagal theory centres on the role of the vagus nerve, the 'wandering nerve' serving the heart, lungs, and digestive tract. Porges hypothesised that there are two vagal systems, a primitive pathway which responds reactively (the freeze response) and a second, more evolved, pathway, which is unique to the mammalian brain, which can draw upon self-regulating behaviours in stressful situations. When trauma occurs beyond the capacity of the evolved system, it shuts down, allowing for the more primitive pathway to take effect. The 'misfiring' or de-inhibition of this vagal system following trauma can be responsible for the hypo/hyper-arousal responses discussed earlier. DMT works from the understanding that the body cyclically responds physically to emotions and then, in turn, emotionally responds to this physical reaction. Introducing body-based grounding techniques that calm this errant vagal system can have a profound impact on the residual effects of trauma and dysregulation. Furthermore, providing clients with concrete actions that rapidly address the enduring impacts of trauma can help challenge perceptions that therapy is too 'intangible' and esoteric to function in the real world.

Accessible examples might include 'peacock breathing' in which a client imagines breathing in and out with the image of a peacock opening and closing its wings. The reader is invited to experience this. You may choose to move more expansively, further opening and expanding your chest with widening arm movements or might move it in miniature tracing the opening and closing patterns with your fingers on your wrists.

This slower, deeper breathing steadies the heartbeat and improves heart rate variability. High heart rate variability is also associated with better emotional regulation, decision-making, and attention. Again, this is a concrete process which the reader can experience simply by resting one hand on their abdomen and another on their heart. Altering the speed of their breath, one can feel the varied rise and fall of their abdomen slowly echoed in the change of heart rate. The vagus nerve is employed in the instinctive process of an infant feeding. This sucking action can be utilised beyond infancy, for example, by giving a client a hard-boiled sweet during moments of hypo/hyper-arousal can re-engage the vagal pathways. The vagus nerve runs along the back of the throat, allowing it to be 'massaged' by deep yogic breathing or the vibrations of chanting or song (Knopik, 2020). This may connect well with populations for whom religious or community events centre on shared noise making. These approaches improve the accessibility of therapy by being body-based, simple techniques. Even transient populations can take these resources with them. There is no cost to breathe.

Conclusion

Accessing adequate mental health support remains a global challenge. By basing our approaches in culturally sensitive, research-informed practice, we can begin to address the difficulties that lie ahead. Our improved understanding of the human brain brings with it the imperative to act in accordance with our knowledge. Neurological research continually strengthens our understanding of the connection between body and mind. DMT is constantly adapting to reflect these changes and improved knowledge. At its core, however, is the universality of movement and the brain that guides it.

Acknowledgements

With the deepest gratitude to Jane Danbold.

With thanks to the organisations which supported me to grow as a therapist, with special recognition to Imara, Dance Movement Therapy Association of Australasia, and Kolkata Sanved.

And with joy for my child, whose first movements were felt alongside these words.

References

Alarcon, R. (2003, February). Mental health and mental health care in Latin America. *World Psychiatry, 2*(1), 54–56. www.ncbi.nlm.nih.gov/pmc/articles/PMC1525063/

Association for Dance Movement Psychotherapy, UK. (2020). https://admp.org.uk

Capello, P. (2016). Looking to the future: Tracking the global emergence of dance/movement therapy. *American Journal of Dance Therapy, 38*(1), 125–138. www.deepdyve.com/lp/springer-journals/looking-to-the-future-tracking-the-global-emergence-of-dance-movement-P0EzXnWyO1?key=springer

Chakraborty, S. (2004). *Kolkata Sanved.* https://kolkatasanved.org/

Danbold, V. (2017). *Moods, moves and mudras.* DTAA Moving On. https://dtaa.org.au/category/2017/vol-14-nos-1-2/

Dance Therapy Association of Australasia. (2017). https://dtaa.org.au

Dickson, C. (2016). Dance under the swastika: Rudolf von Laban's influence on Nazi power. *International Journal of Undergraduate Research and Creative Activities, 8*(1), 7. http://doi.org/10.7710/2168-0620.1063

Eberhard-Kaechele, M. (2012). Memory, metaphor and mirroring in movement therapy with trauma. Chp. 17. In S. Koch et al. (Eds.), *John Benjamins publishing company.* https://books.google.co.uk/books?id=IaovW-rP-RcC&1pg=PA267&dq=mirroring%20dance%20movement%20therapy&lr&pg=PP1#v=onepage&q=mirroring%20dance%20movement%20therapy&f=false

Felitti, V. J., Anda, R. F., Nordenberg, D., Williamson, D. F., Spitz, A. M., Edwards, V., Koss, M. P., & Marks, J. S. (1998). Relationship of childhood abuse and household dysfunction to many of the leading causes of death in adults. The adverse childhood experiences (ACE) study. *American Journal of Preventive Medicine, 14*(4), 245–258. doi:10.1016/s0749-3797(98)00017-8. PMID: 9635069. https://pubmed.ncbi.nlm.nih.gov/9635069/

Funk, M., Lund, C., & Drew, N. (2013–2020). *Mental health, human rights & legislation.* www.who.int/mental_health/policy/legislation/en/

Garfinkel, Y. (2011). *Dance in prehistoric Europe.* www.researchgate.net/publication/270031029_Dance_in_Prehistoric_Europe

Gendlin, E. T. (1981). Movement therapy, objectification, and focusing. *The Focusing Folio, 1*(2), 35–37. http://previous.focusing.org/gendlin/docs/gol_2016.html

Gupta, S., & Mittal, S. (2013, January–June). Yawning and its physiological significance. *International Journal of Applied and Basic Medical Research, 3*(1), 11–15. www.ncbi.nlm.nih.gov/pmc/articles/PMC3678674/

Iacoboni, M., & Depratto, M. (2006). The mirror neuron system and the consequences of its dysfunction. *Nature Reviews Neuroscience, 7*, 942–951. www.nature.com/articles/nrn2024?r=1&l=ri&fst=0

Kim, S., Fonagy, P., Allen, J., & Strathearn, L. (2014). Mothers' unresolved trauma blunts amygdala response to infant distress. *Society for Neuroscience, 9*(4), 352–336. www.ncbi.nlm.nih.gov/pmc/articles/PMC4260525/

Kinouani, G. (2017). *Culturally biased therapy? (Part 1) epistemic violence and CBT.* https://racereflections.co.uk/culturally-biased-therapy-epistemic-violence-and-cbt

Knopik, V. (2020). *Polyvagal theory and breath.* https://yogadigest.com/polyvagal-theory-and-the-breath/

Koch, S., & Fischman, D. (2011). Embodied enactive dance/movement therapy. *American Journal of Dance Therapy, 33*(1), 57–72. https://link.springer.com/article/10.1007/s10465-011-9108-4

Loman, S. (2016). Judith S. Kestenberg's dance/movement therapy legacy: Approaches with pregnancy, young children, and caregivers. *American Journal of Dance Therapy, 38*(2), 225–244.

Loman, S., & Foley, L. (1996). Model for understanding the nonverbal process in relationships. *The Arts in Psychotherapy, 23*(4), 341–350.

Mastrominico, A., Fuchs, T., Manders, E., Steffinger, L., Hirjak, D., Sieber, M., Thomas, E., Holzinger, A., Konrad, A., Bopp, N., & Koch, S. C. (2018). Effects of dance movement therapy on adult patients with autism spectrum disorder: A randomized controlled trial. *Behavioural Sciences, 8*(7), 61. www.ncbi.nlm.nih.gov/pmc/articles/PMC6071290/

McNeil, W. (2009). *Keeping together in time: Dance and drill in human history.* https://books.google.co.uk/books?id=4XLBfff6VnsC&lpg=PP1&dq=inauthor%3A%22William%20Hardy%20MCNEILL%22&hl=de&pg=PP1#v=&q&=false

McNeil, W. (2020.). *Muscular bonding: How dance made us human.* https://fs.blog/2020/04/muscular-bonding/

Ogden, P., & Minton, K. (2000). *Sensorimotor psychotherapy: One method for processing traumatic memory.* https://doi.org/10.1177/153476560000600302

Payne, H. (Ed.). (1992). *Dance/movement therapy: Theory and practice.* Routledge.

Porges, S. (1994). *Home of Dr Stephen Porges.* www.stephenporges.com

Psychological Health and Wellness Clinic. (2021). https://phwcbd.org

Schulte-Rüther, M., Otte, E., Adigüzel, K., Firk, C., Herpertz-Dahlmann, B., Koch, I., & Konrad, K. (2016). *Intact mirror mechanisms for automatic facial emotions in children and adolescents with autism spectrum disorder.* https://onlinelibrary.wiley.com/doi/full/10.1002/aur.1654

Sharma, I. (2020). *Living in chains.* www.hrw.org/report/2020/10/06/living-chains/shackling-people-psychosocial-disabilities-worldwide

Siegel, D. J. (1999). *The developing mind.* Guilford Press.

Song, S. (2009). *Does famine influence sex ratio at birth? Evidence from the 1959–1961 great leap forward famine in China.* www.ncbi.nlm.nih.gov/pmc/articles/PMC3367790/

Tosey, P. (1992). The snake sheds a skin theme of order and chaos in dance movement therapy. Chp. 12. In H. Payne (Ed.). *Dance movement therapy: Theory and practice.* Tavistock and Routledge.

UNESCO Institute for Statistics. (2018). *One in five children, adolescents and youth is out of school.* http://uis.unesco.org/en/news/education-data-release-one-every-five-children-adolescents-and-youth-out-school

Wittbrodt, M. T., Moazzami, K., Lima, B. B., Alam, Z. S., Corry, D., Hammadah, M., Campanella, C., Ward, L., Quyyumi, A. A., Shah, A. J., Vaccarino, V., Nye, J. A., & Douglas Bremner, J. (2019, July). Early childhood trauma alters neurological responses to mental stress in patients with coronary artery disease. *Journal of Affective Disorders, 254,* 49–58. https://pubmed.ncbi.nlm.nih.gov/31103906/

World Health Organization (WHO). (2019). *Autism spectrum disorders.* www.who.int/news-room/fact-sheets/detail/autism-spectrum-disorders

York, K. (2020). *BAME representation and psychology.* https://thepsychologist.bps.org.uk/volume-33/january-2020/bame-representation-and-psychology

Youssef, N., Lockwood, L., Su, S., Hao, G., & Rutton, B. (2018). The effects of trauma, with or without PTSD, on the transgenerational DNA methylation alterations in human offspring. *Brain Sciences, 8*(5), 83. doi:10.3390/brainsci8050083

Part III

Reflections and review

12 Reflections

Caroline Miller

As editors of this volume, we are hoping that this is the first of many. We hope that future volumes will continue with the marriage of the arts therapies and neurosciences and that they will involve writers from an even wider collection of countries and with a wider range of ethnic voices. We can see, in writing this book, that the necessity to use English creates biases in writing and publishing, in much of the world, towards UK and US trainings and their offshoots. We also see that the dominant styles of academic writing demand that intuitive cultural responses may be lost in translation. Nevertheless, this book makes a start with a small but diverse collection of countries, writers, and practices.

Writers in this book were asked to look at their practice through the lenses of the arts therapies and neuroscience and to indicate how these two disciplines work together in a variety of situations. They were asked to find appropriate ways to track changes observed with clients through therapeutic sessions, which could be used in research projects or in daily practice with clients. They were asked to provide examples from their practices and the settings in which they worked with clients. These simple guidelines unearthed a world of riches.

The key element in all psychotherapies is to be safely, professionally, and kindly alongside our clients as they need us to be. This is so that they feel safe enough and in a relationship which allows them to do their work. This book reaffirms the foundational principle of the psychological therapies, that the most important element in any effective therapy is the therapeutic relationship. This is supported by neuroscience which provides the physical and theoretical basis for why this is important and how it works through our bodies and minds and behaviours in any of our approaches. Neuroscience reaffirms our common humanity, with our need to have feelings and dilemmas heard, understood, and taken seriously. Neuroscience, along with knowledge of human development in its wider forms, offers us new understandings of how we work as arts therapists and why arts therapies are effective. It shows us that having an awareness of underlying neurological development and neuroscience can enhance our work and help us make greater sense of our interactions with our clients and of their responses to us.

In the arts therapies, we often speak of the triangular relationship which exists with the therapist and the client as two aspects of the triangle, with the

DOI: 10.4324/9781003082897-17

third being the arts modality. The arts modality connects the therapist and client and, at the same time, brings direct involvement with, and communication through, an arts medium. Music therapy, dance movement therapy, drama therapy, and art therapy all involve embodiment, increased physical activity, and choices to be made in the immediate environment among materials to be used, interactions to enter or decline, responses made to stimulating materials, activities, and often to other people. The materials on offer provide a range of textures and colours, stories, and games and structured and unstructured movement, and sound can provide alternative communication methods to speech. Arts therapies also provide whole-body and mind engagement at the same time as stimulating creativity and imagination. These can be modulated to match developmental stages and, especially with a knowledge of neuroscience, can help therapists to recognise where trauma or neglect have interrupted neurological and related development so they can target reparative therapy to those stages. Creative work stimulates creative responses and new ways to approach old problems. The arts therapies are grounded in the reality and physicality of our bodies and minds which all humans share. With backing from neuroscience, they are grounded in clearly observed connections between our minds and bodies, between our actions and reactions, and between the impact of neglectful or traumatic experiences which have a direct impact on the brain and on subsequent behaviour.

The arts therapies, and other psychotherapies, do not work by magic but by processes (regardless of the theoretical orientation of the therapist) which are observable and traceable, with findings from neuroscience. Therapy is not a process of magic, but moments in therapy and therapeutic outcomes can be quite magical. Each of these writers has illustrated both moments of magic and magical outcomes, with arts therapy and scientific approaches married to the best interests of their clients.

The creativity of arts therapists helps them find and adapt creative approaches. Examples from writers in this book include adapting community choir models for therapeutic effect and finding a compatible research method to studying the effect of special groups singing in special choirs; adapting the Men's Shed model within a hospice setting; using research methods that suit the particular communities involved; using familiar movement patterns to bring together representatives of many countries in readiness for political and social discussions to address common issues in those countries; developing Narradrama from dramatherapy and then Narradrama as a Three Act Play, complete with using a range of research methods to fit a particular client group; and utilising dance and movement with groups experiencing social and mental health problems. All of these are a long way from notions of therapy involving only talk and only occurring between therapist and client/s.

Cathy Malchiodi has written extensively about the creative arts therapies (sometimes as expressive therapies) as combinations of dance/movement, music, drama, sand play therapy, poetry and writing therapy, and other arts, as effective in various situations particularly in the treatment of trauma. The combinations of arts therapies may have exponential effects in therapy with some people. Malchiodi (2005) writes that "[o]ne individual may be more visual, another more tactile, and so forth. When therapists are able to include these various expressive capacities in their work with clients, they can more fully enhance each person's abilities to communicate effectively and authentically" (p. 1).

In 2012 she writes "the relationship between neuroscience and art therapy is an important one that influences every area of practice" (Malchiodi, 2012, p. 17). This is followed by a description of creative arts therapies and brain-wide approaches to therapy with attachment focus (Malchiodi, 2013) and with trauma-informed therapy which integrates neurodevelopmental knowledge and the sensory qualities of the arts in trauma work.

Neuroscience-informed therapy places neuroscience on an equal footing with the arts therapies, not in a hierarchy in which science seems more important or to carry more weight.

Arts therapists do not have access to the technology that neuroscientists have. They do not want it or need it because they can call on neuroscience research. Similarly, they can liaise with arts therapists' observations of behaviours and changes to align with some of their own.

All the writers in this book have assumed the roles of therapists, creative artists, writers, academics, and researchers as they have written stories of arts therapies to share with a wider group of readers. They have all been open to new ideas and new constructions of how to view their work. Connections with neuroscientific findings have amplified their own understanding of their work. We hope that reading these accounts will do the same for the readers.

References

Malchiodi, C. (2005). Expressive therapies history, theory and practice. Chp 1. In C. Malchiodi (Ed.), *Expressive therapies*. Guilford Publications.

Malchiodi, C. (2012). Art therapy and the brain. In C. Malchiodi (Ed.), *Handbook of art therapy* (pp. 17–26). Guilford Press.

Malchiodi, C. (2013). *Creative art therapy and attachment work.* https://www.psychologytoday.com/us/blog/arts-and-health/201309/creative-art-therapy-and-attachment-work

13 Future developments

Caroline Miller and Mariana Torkington

This chapter offers a final reflection that looks forward to future developments in theory and practice in the arts therapies.

The group of writers represented in this book set out to honour their clients' stories through the use of expressive therapies and, in doing so, have paved the way for further innovation in the field. The expressive or creative therapies have been gaining wider recognition in the past few decades. Phil Jones (2021) stated that a growing number of people are again seeking an arts therapy approach to treatment. He proposed that the arts therapies should continue to develop understandings of the relations among theory, research, and practice and highlighted a series of interviews with a focus on research in the arts therapies around the world.

We propose that wider collaboration in the arts therapies will facilitate innovation in these areas and contribute to the health and well-being of our global communities. We anticipate that there would be interest in learning about the work conducted by indigenous arts therapists, and expressive arts therapists throughout Asia, South America, and other regions, where ongoing research and practice with diverse populations may be under-reported.

Overall, it has been reassuring and exciting to see how findings from neuroscience support the theory and practice of the arts therapies. Things we have done for years now have an additional rationale for their use and a greater understanding of why they are so effective. Other approaches which have inexplicably not worked so well can be re-examined through a neuroscience and developmental lens and adjusted creatively. Neuroscience does not dictate the practice of the arts therapies, but it has a great deal to add to our understanding of our practice and our clients.

Looking to the future we hope for greater liaison and learning between the arts therapies and neurosciences; and for more prolific publication of increased research in the arts therapies using a variety of research methods. We may not find it appropriate to use some of the more traditional scientific research methods, but we can certainly learn from scientific research and rigorous approaches. We hope that arts therapists will find inspiration in seeing ever more clearly how their clients respond and what they respond to. For many years there has been a false divide between the arts and the sciences, with venerable arts

DOI: 10.4324/9781003082897-18

therapists like Frances Kaplan (2000, art therapist and chemist) devoting much of their writing to bringing arts and sciences into closer alignment. Neuroscientists have not (yet) been able to locate the soul or the spirit or intuition, but many scientific discoveries have relied on that moment of sudden realisation to bring years of work to fruition. Maybe scientific Eureka moments and therapist intuition have a lot in common.

Moon and Hoffman (2014) have written about art-based research innovation in graduate art therapy education and contend that art-based research "offers a valuable alternative to academic expectations that presume that the best means to demonstrate mastery of learning is by completing a social science research project that results in a traditional thesis" (p. 1). McNiff (1998) suggested that arts therapists "need to use their artistic sensibilities in the practice of inquiry" (p. 11). Our book and those of our colleagues in the arts therapies around the world indicate the need for further collaboration across all the expressive therapies (art, dance and movement, drama, and music therapy) to find intersecting points of learning and practice.

We put this book together during a global pandemic. We are still living through this, with greater degrees of difficulty and grief being experienced in some countries than in others. However, we are all affected personally, socially, and politically. All of us, in every country, experienced long periods of isolation and restriction as COVID-19 became a central focus for humanity. This experience is unprecedented for current generations, with an impact on people from all walks of life and social and economic status. Arts therapists showed great resilience, along with most of humanity, during this period. Perhaps the pandemic has also delivered to humanity an opportunity for greater 'enforced reflection' on what it means to be human. Porges (2020) spoke about the impact of COVID-19 on the psychotherapeutic community and on our clients, addressing our contradictory needs for social engagement and social distancing. He also signalled that 'our nervous system wants to connect with others', a need that is thwarted by the challenges associated with COVID-19 throughout the world. Perhaps this is a time in our history when we pause to think about our social, emotional, and psychological needs and attend to our humanity in all its manifestations.

We propose that this is a time for us, collectively, to move assertively towards more holistic forms of treatment that address the physical, mental, emotional, social, cultural, and spiritual needs of our clients. There are examples in these chapters. This approach could be reflected in the training provided by tertiary institutions through a variety of research methods, attention to areas of emerging interest and value such as neuroscience and addressing human development training and ecological models of writing and teaching. There is a growing need to learn more about the use of virtual technology as this is likely to become more necessary for arts therapies practice in the future (Liu & Chang, 2018). Those expanding needs may sometimes clash with our wider respect for the earth and nature, as we have seen what disasters can occur on a global scale, at the same time as we have experienced increases in bird and animal life with the reduction in traffic, environmental noise, and other environmental pollution.

We need to continue to learn from those like Porges (2020), Schore (2000), and Siegel (2012), who have paved the way in refusing to accept a split between mind and body and have demonstrated how the effects of trauma and anxiety, for example, can be modified by physical movement and breathing. Just as COVID-19 has brought focus to our common humanity, we can look to our common, and different, professional approaches, sharing and learning from all the arts therapies and from other professions.

Above all, we can stay hopeful and creative in our own lives, in our work with clients, and in research and writing about our work. In COVID-19 times we find ourselves, globally, dealing with the psychological impact of pain and suffering. With mental health crises in most countries exacerbated by unequal access to mental health and other health treatment, arts therapies have much to offer.

As humanity finds itself dealing with these difficult times, we can take some comfort in the knowledge that creativity is an innate human function which can provide hope, inspiration, and solutions to the problems that confront us and our clients in our daily lives. We need creativity in all its forms more than ever, and we believe that by tapping into creativity and its associated functions of intuition and imagination, that we can move together towards a different world and a greater capacity for human generosity and sharing.

References

Jones, P. (2021). *The arts therapies a revolution in healthcare*. Routledge.

Kaplan, F. (2000). *Art, science and art therapy repainting the future*. Jessica Kingsley.

Liu, Y., & Chang, C. (2018). *The application of virtual reality technology in art therapy: A case of tilt brush*. 1st IEEE International Conference on Knowledge Innovation and Invention, Taiwan. https://ieeexplore.ieee.org/xpl/conhome/8543366/proceeding

McNiff, S. (1998). *Art-based research*. Jessica Kingsley.

Moon, B. L., & Hoffman, N. (2014). Performing art-based research: Innovation in graduate art therapy education. *Art Therapy: Journal of the American Art Therapy Association, 31*(4), 172–178.

Porges, S. (2020). *COVID-19 anxiety, cultivating safeness, and polyvagal theory with Dr. Stephen Porges*. Psychologists Off the Clock. Apple Music Podcast. https://podcasts.apple.com/us/podcast/covid-19-anxiety-cultivating-safeness-polyvagal-theory/id1176171178?i=1000468482088

Schore, A. N. (2000). Attachment and the regulation of the right brain. *Attachment and Human Development, 2*(1), 23–47.

Siegel, D. (2012). Mind, brain and relationships. The interpersonal neurobiology perspective. In D. Siegel (Ed.), *The developing mind. How relationships and the brain interact to shape who we are* (2nd ed., p. 66). Guilford Press.

Index

Page numbers in *italics* indicate a figure on the corresponding page.